SPIRITS WITH
SCALPELS

To:

Eleanor
Jennifer
David
Suzanne

With whom I am grateful to have shared this lifetime.

SPIRITS WITH SCALPELS

THE CULTURALBIOLOGY OF RELIGIOUS HEALING IN BRAZIL

SIDNEY M. GREENFIELD

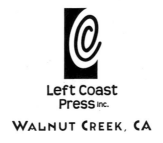

Left Coast
Press inc.

WALNUT CREEK, CA

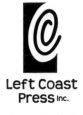

Left Coast Press, Inc.
1630 North Main Street, #400
Left Coast
Press Inc.
Walnut Creek, California 94596
http://www.lcoastpress.com

Hardback ISBN 978-1-59874-367-8
Paperback ISBN 978-1-59874-368-5

Library of Congress Cataloging in Publication Data Available

09 10 11 5 4 3

Printed in the United States of America

⊖™ The paper used in this publication meets the minimum requirements of American National Standard for Information Sciences—Permanence of Paper for Printed Library Materials, ANSI/NISO Z39.48—1992.

Cover art by Margo Magid; cover design by Hannah Jennings.

Chapters 1, 2, and 3 include materials previously published in "The Return of Dr. Fritz: Spiritist Healing and Patronage Networks in Urban, Industrial Brazil." *Social Science and Medicine* 24(1987):1095-1108.

Parts of Chapter 4 appeared in "The Patients of Dr. Fritz: Assessments of Treatment by a Brazilian Spiritist Healer." *Journal of the Society for Psychical Research* 61(1997):372-383.

Chapter 5 is a revision and modification of "Chapter 6, 'A Transiçãode Miguel Müller: A Doença, a Cura e a Morte com Dignidade de uma Racionalista Secular no Brasil Meridional,'" in *Cirugias do Além: Pesquisas Antropológicas Sobre Curas Espirituais.* Sidney M. Greenfield. Petrópolis, RJ: Editora Vozes, 1999:169-91.

Chapter 6 is a revision and adaptation of materials that previously appeared in "Treating the Sick with a Morality Play: The Kardecist-Spiritist Disobession in Brazil." *Social Analysis* 48(2004):2:174-194; "Legacies from the Past and Transitions to a 'Healed' Future in Brazilian Spiritist Therapy." *Anthropologica* 35(1993):23-38; and "Spirits and Spiritist Therapy in Southern Brazil: A Case Study of an Innovative, Syncretic Healing Group." *Culture, Medicine and Psychiatry* 16(1992):23-51.

Chapter 9 is adapted from "Pilgrimage Healing in Northeast Brazil: A Culturalbiological Explanation." *Pilgrimage and Healing,* edited by Jill Dubisch and Michael Winkelman. Tuscon, AZ: University of Arizona Press, 2005: 3-23; and "Pilgrimage and Patronage in Brazil: A Paradigm for Social Relations and Religious Diversity." *Luso-Brazilian Review* 43:2(2006):63-87 (both with Antonio Mourão Cavalcante).

Parts of Chapter 10 appeared in "Descendants of European Immigrants in Southern Brazil as Participants and Heads of Afro-Brazilian Religious Centers." *Ethnic and Racial Studies* 17:4(1994):684-700.

Chapter 15 contains materials previously published in "Recovering and Reconstructing Syncretism." *Reinventing Religions: Syncretism and Transformation in Africa and the Americas.* edited by Sidney M. Greenfield and André Droogers. Lanham, MD: Rowman and Littlefield Publishers, Inc, 2001: 21-42.

Chapter 16 is adapted and modified from "The Culturalbiology of Brazilian Spiritist Surgery and Other Non-Biomedical Healing." *International Journal of Parapsychology* 13(2002-2005): [forthcoming].

CONTENTS

PROLOGUE

A study in the July 11, 2002, issue of the *New England Journal of Medicine* reported that many patients who received only simulated surgery on their arthritic knees did as well as, and at times better than, the group who were the subjects of actual surgical interventions. Patients who received placebo surgery experienced less pain. Their knees functioned better for two years following incisions simulating arthroscopic surgery. No cartilage was actually removed.[1]

Placebo surgery?

Although critics have raised questions about who was selected for the treatment, that doesn't affect my own special interest in the results. I'm delighted by yet another professional, "scientific" demonstration in this country of the power of surgical interventions to produce what patients experience as improvement in their conditions, even when the work of the scalpel has nothing to do with treatment as understood by mainstream Western medicine.

Over a period of more than two and one-half decades in Brazil I witnessed and videotaped scores of "surgeries" in which Spiritist healer-mediums, most lacking any professional medical credentials, cut into their patients, sometimes in extraordinary ways, to achieve results that large numbers considered successful. What would the authors of the knee study and their critics think of what I saw and learned?

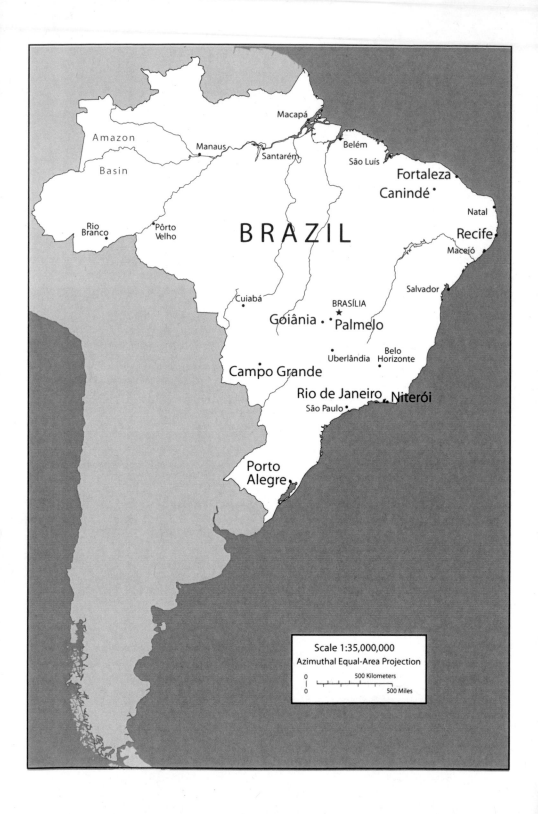

AN INVITATION AND INTRODUCTION

I would like to invite the reader to join me on an adventure to a land where spirits, incorporated in mediums, cut into patients with scalpels, kitchen knives, and even electric saws to remove, at times with unwashed fingers, infected materials and growths. Yet the patients are given no anesthetic, feel little if any pain, and develop no infections. They recover without complications. People suffering from physical and emotional symptoms participate in rituals in which specialists enter into trances, incorporating antagonists from patients' previous lifetimes. The antagonists are talked into stopping whatever they are doing that is causing the problem. When they do, the suffering party recovers. Still other people go on pilgrimages, traveling sometimes hundreds of miles on foot to visit the shrine of a saint to pay a debt incurred for recovery from a broken limb, cancer, or some other illness. Alternatively, a patient, after being mysteriously cured of symptoms that a doctor may not have been able to diagnose, thanks a deity from Africa, embodied in a host, or the spirit of a deceased rogue, prostitute, or slave, and becomes an initiate in a religion whose origins go back to villages in West Africa from which the ancestors of slaves were taken centuries ago. Some people accept Jesus and join a Pentecostal church after being inexplicably cured of their symptoms by the Holy Ghost following prayer by a pastor speaking in tongues.

Our trip is to Brazil, the largest of the nations in South America, but we will not be going for carnival, attending a soccer match, dancing sambas, or seeing Corcovado, the majestic statue of Christ overlooking beautiful Guanabara Bay. We will not be going to the Amazon to experience the forest that is so important for the maintenance of the global environment, to explore its thousands of different plants and animals, to fish for piranhas, or to meet Indians. Instead, our itinerary will take us to urban centers where most of the country's 185 million people live. Here we will meet ordinary folk: beauticians, bank clerks, businessmen, policewomen, students, agricultural workers, lawyers, university professors, doctors, the unemployed, preachers, spirit mediums, the rich, the poor, people of all races and classes.

When they are sick, Brazilians seek traditional medicine. Should they not recover, they turn to spirits or other supernatural beings postulated in the worldviews of diverse religious groups in competition with each other for members. Each group preaches a compelling narrative of the spiritual and emotional benefits to be gained by those who accept the truths of its particular view of the cosmos. The help of the supernatural(s) with problems of this world is a further inducement to join. We will observe how the sick and suffering go about choosing a religious group, affiliate with it when their symptoms disappear, or seek a different group when they do not. Some people leave a group, perhaps only recently joined, when it does not provide them with relief during a second emergency. As a result, different members of one family or household might belong to different religions. The general pattern resulting from this array of decisions and choices made by Brazilians in search of healing will be referred to as a religious marketplace.

The central problem we will attempt to resolve is how to explain the recoveries. Those who provide the treatment attribute recovery to the supernatural(s) of their religious traditions. Medical science disagrees. The events are considered anomalies in the paradigms of the sciences that inform it. Must we accept the contentions of the religious leaders for our explanation? Can science be adapted to explain the events? This dilemma places us at the interface of religion and science.

Your participation is under the direction of an anthropologist. Contrary to what is taught today, I learned and still believe that anthropology "is the interrelation of what is biological in man[2] and what is social and historical in him" (Kroeber [1921] 1948:2). Until my senior year in college, I did not even know anthropology existed. Required to take an introductory course in anthropology to complete my studies in economics and sociology, I was fascinated to realize that there were people in the world who thought, felt, behaved, and made decisions based on assumptions different than those of the people I knew growing up. My instructor suggested that I continue my studies at Columbia University, where all graduate students in the anthropology program were required to take a year-long course that offered an overview of the four fields basic to the discipline: physical anthropology (or human biology), archaeology, linguistics, and cultural anthropology. I also enrolled in a class offered by Professor Charles Wagley, the department chair, who was a well-respected specialist in Brazilian studies. I was hooked on the first day and decided that this was where I wanted to do research.

One of my teachers was Margaret Mead. Her words orient my lifelong fascination as a professional anthropologist. Mead said in class and wrote, "Anthropology demands the open-mindedness with which one must look and listen, record in astonishment and wonder at that which one would not have been able to guess." To this she added that we should examine critically all the knowledge brought together by our academic colleagues to explain what we find among peoples from other cultural traditions.

In my first research, on the island of Barbados, I was part of a group of scholars and students trying to apply the ethnographic techniques developed in the study of small-scale marginal peoples, such as Melanesian Islanders, African tribes, and American Indians, to peoples in more complex societies. My research was on family and kinship, but we were living in a small village of descendants of African slaves whose survival still depended on the production of sugar. I wondered: How did the world of plantations and African slavery that dominated the history of the tropical New World come into being?

It was to take two and a half decades for me to get to Portugal and the island of Madeira to examine fifteenth-century archival documents to find the answer. This reading about the Portuguese expansion in the fifteenth and sixteenth centuries informs my understanding of the early colonization of Brazil.

The southern part of the state of Minas Gerais, a region known to be politically conservative and very traditional, was the site of my first Brazilian research in 1959. I collaborated with the resident sociologist, who also was a politician and attorney, on a study of patronage and politics. The hierarchical nature of Brazilian society and the importance of relations of patronage and dependency became a key factor in my future research.

I was fortunate to become a professional anthropologist in the half century following World War II, when the United States was expanding economically and engaged in world affairs. Money for research related to development was available, and I was able to design my studies to qualify for this funding. Thus I was able to do work that provided background for my present research.

In 1981, while in the city of Fortaleza in the Brazilian northeast, I encountered the first of several Spiritist healer-mediums. For the next twenty seven years, the interface of science and religion were to consume me.

The first time I witnessed a Spiritist surgery I could not believe my eyes. A young man named José Carlos Ribeiro took a used scalpel from a tray that I was holding and plunged it into the eye of an elderly man. The patient did not move, other than to swat away a fly, when the healer levered the eye out of its socket. Sometime later, when I observed Edson Queiroz slice into an unanesthetized woman's breast and then insert his bloodstained fingers into the opening to tear out a tumor, my disbelief escalated. Years after that, as Antonio de Oliveira Rios, with the dirty blade of an electrical saw, cut into the spine of a young man who had lost the use of his legs after a gunshot wound (and, like the others, had been given no anesthetic), I still was not able to comprehend what I was seeing. Besides the challenge of explaining these perplexing events, I was concerned that no one would believe me when I told them about it. Both problems were exacerbated when I viewed ritual activities during which African-derived deities and a variety of other supernatural entities, incorporated in the bodies of adepts of Candomblé, Umbanda, Pentecostalism, and other popular Brazilian religions, provided therapies that participants, like the surgical patients, claimed had cured them of a variety of conditions. Subsequently, I used a video camera, not just to document the phenomenon for colleagues, students, and skeptics, but also to make several films of the surgeries and other therapeutic ritual practices (see Greenfield 1995; Greenfield and Gray 1989, 1988, 1985). The still photographs found throughout this book were excerpted from these videos.

Observing these events, and following their effects on patients, forced me to question almost everything I had ever learned about healing and the practice of medicine and surgery. Growing up in the United States, I accepted biomedical practices routinely. But in Brazil I witnessed forms of therapy that could not be explained in terms of scientific medicine. How could patients who were not given anything to prevent pain be cut into and not experience pain, as they have reported so often? Why didn't they develop infections or other complications when operated on with unclean instruments? Could uneducated and untrained individuals, as many of the healers are, perform surgeries or prescribe medications and not do harm to those they treat? Moreover, why would people seek out and submit themselves to such unusual treatments? Was this not the essence of the interrelation between biology and culture?

I use the term *culture* in the broad, holistic, and integrative sense first proposed by Sir Edward B. Tylor ([1871] 1958) in the late nineteenth century and employed so insightfully by practitioners on both sides of the Atlantic Ocean in the first three-quarters of the twentieth century. I modify his usage to follow Geertz's (1973) emphasis on the systems of symbolic meanings that human beings learn when they are born into a specific community and use to orient their understandings of themselves and the situations in which they find themselves. In this view, human beings are seen, in Max Weber's sense, as animals suspended in webs of significance they themselves have spun.

Weber's generally cited usage is modified to emphasize that it is not independent, single persons who, on their own, form the meanings that orient their behavior, but rather that individuals use and respond to what they have learned by virtue of being born and socialized in a specific time and place. Individuals may modify what they have learned from those around them and from previous generations. In this way, meaning systems are not created out of whole cloth by the efforts or agency of specific persons, but rather are the products of the interactions of multiple parties in social situations that are shared and passed on to the next generation. This usage permits us to explore social processes to include "a tissue of relationships between man as biological entity and the unique structure of symbols and techniques that [enable him to adapt to his environment and] results in maintaining his existence" (Polanyi, Arensberg, and Pearson 1957:239). Moreover, the content of the meaning systems orients the decisions and choices made in the many and diverse situations people encounter in the course of their daily lives. These outcomes produce the patterns of behavior whose observation and description constitute the essence of ethnography (Greenfield and Strickon 1981).

Culture, thus understood, makes it possible to examine how the meaning systems adhered to and shared by members of a given society—or segment in a complex one—interface with, influence, and are influenced by the organic systems and processes of the members of the group. How this affects organs, molecules, and genes in what we are calling culturalbiology is paramount to the analysis. We can examine how the symbols of the belief system of a group, which may be expressed explicitly or held implicitly as assumptions, inform decision making and, for our purposes, interrelate with the biology of those who live in terms of the meanings and beliefs.

Our journey takes us to the laboratories and offices of researchers and clinicians working at the forefront of modern medicine to examine the assumptions on which the practice of medicine is based and how these assumptions are being reformulated to bring together in a single view the opposition previously made between body and mind. We will explore the similarities between the content of the suggestions used in hypnotically facilitated therapy and symbolic beliefs such as those held by each of Brazil's popular religions. Both offer directions intended to help an afflicted individual exposed to them recover. This imagery, based on communication and information flow, enables us to see, in a new way, "the interrelation of what is biological in man and what is social and [cultural] in him" (Kroeber [1921] 1948:2).

What has developed into this book began as an article about the Spiritist surgeries that Warner Bloomberg Jr. and I drafted for submission to a popular magazine. The article was never published, primarily because the editor found the content too unbelievable. I have revised that manuscript, some of which forms part of the first four

chapters. I am most grateful to Professor Bloomberg for his contribution and the impetus he provided for this project.

Consistent with the approach Bloomberg and I used in drafting
the article, there is much more of me included in the descriptions of
Spiritist healers and surgeries in these chapters than I usually include
in my ethnographic writings. I trust that the reader will not find
more of the author than necessary in the first section.

We start at Brazilian religious centers and examine the many varied traditions and their histories in the country. Spiritism is introduced and the therapeutic treatments offered by healer-mediums are
described. The discussion and analysis of the belief system are included in the form of "asides" as the actions of the healer-mediums and
their patients are chronicled. These asides contain what in anthropology is called the emic explanation for the events (Pike 1967).
The first three chapters concentrate on specific healer-mediums and
their patients during the 1980s. The healer-mediums are José Carlos Ribeiro in Fortaleza; Edson Queiroz in Recife; and Antonio de
Oliveira Rios in Palmelo. Chapter 4 describes treatments by Mauricio Magalhães and the follow-up survey of his patients conducted
in Campo Grande in the early 1990s. Spiritist healers do not cure all
their patients; what happens when they do not is presented in chapter 5. The case study of the death of my friend and colleague Paulo
Schutz is detailed to explain such an event. Chapter 6 on disobsessions, a uniquely Karadecist form of noninvasive therapy, follows.
This section ends with the spirit of Dr. Fritz, while incorporated in
Edson Queiroz, explaining why he actually cuts into patients when
according to the belief system it is not necessary. His goal is to pro-
voke those he treats, and observers, by making them think about the
inexplicable surgeries, and in the end to convert them to the Spiritist
belief system. A further examination of similar practices by Brazil's
other faiths, and their attempts to attract new members in the competitive religious marketplace, follows.

In part II, beginning in chapter 8, we look at other "popular"
Brazilian religions, with a brief history of religious diversity. Their
respective meaning systems—theologies—are examined in descriptions of their healing practices, providing a series of alternative emic
explanations for therapeutic practices. Chapter 9 takes us on a pilgrimage to the shrine of St. Francis of Assisi in the northeastern

municipality of Canindé during its annual festival. "Popular" Catholicism, the predominant form the religion took in Brazil over much of its history, is shown to be the exemplar on which the others are modeled. Most pilgrims who participate in the ritual journey do so to discharge an obligation incurred when they first asked the saint to intercede and help them to be cured of an illness. The African traditions brought to Brazil by slaves, and their adaptation to the national religious scene, are examined in chapter 10. A case study of Umbanda, demonstrating how its intentionally created supernatural pantheon, working through mediums, provides healing and helps the needy in an attempt to gain followers, is presented in chapter 11. Chapter 12 turns to evangelical Protestantism, particularly Pentecostalism, the fastest growing religion in Brazil, if not the world. Chapter 13 explores the social, demographic, and economic transformations of the second half of the twentieth century that provide the background needed for understanding the contest for followers by the competing faiths. It concludes with a model of how popular religions in Brazil interrelate with each other as competitors for the same pool of potential worshippers. It is within this marketplace, characterized by reciprocity, that religious groups offer the help of their supernatural(s) in exchange for affiliation and devotion from those who shop for assistance.

From the perspective of the sociology of Brazilian religion, this chapter summarizes what I believe to be one of the more important contributions of the book. While I might have begun with the presentation of a model of the reciprocal exchange of gifts in the religious marketplace—derived from Polanyi's economic analysis of trade and markets (Polanyi, Arensberg, and Pearson 1957)—and then presented the descriptive materials to illustrate it, I chose instead to present the descriptive materials first, in part because they are so compelling but more importantly because as an empiricist I prefer to let models emerge from data.

Part III moves from the sociology of Brazilian religion back to the search for a scientific explanation for the medically anomalous variety of treatments described. I rejected parapsychology and other epistemological alternatives to science from the outset and assumed instead that an explanation might be found within the framework of conventional medicine and the science that informs it. Seeking the interrelation between culture and biology, approaches to healing that question the still widely held Cartesian dualism that opposes mind and body are explored.

Immunology investigates the role the immune system plays in the prevention and cure of illness. Research describing how social and psychological factors (psychobiology) contribute to the weakening of that system and lead to the onset of some diseases attracted my attention. While exploring these alternative therapies, I was impressed by clinicians who stimulate the immune systems of patients using a variety of therapeutic techniques and succeed in diminishing the manifestations of illness.[3]

The developing field of psychoneuroimmunology, which combines psychotherapy and physiological immunology, added a further dimension to my search. The successful use of hypnosis by some psychotherapists directed me to study, and then undergo training in, hypnosis and hypnotherapy.

While we read daily of efforts to formulate epistemological systems that will integrate the proliferation of these ideas and theories in the field of health and medicine, this work is still in its early stages. Hence what I offer is, at best, tentative. I have attempted to place this growing body of research within a cultural framework by reintroducing the symbolic meaning dimension of beliefs, conceptualized as information in a communications model of human illness and healing. One of my hopes is to propose future directions for research and perhaps some brave new ideas.

How healing by spirits has been treated in the anthropological literature, by tracing the discussion back to the time when science split from religion, is found in chapter 14. The position taken, and still held by many contemporary scholars, is based on the thinking of the French philosopher René Descartes. When he opposed mind and body in an attempt to create an independent domain for science, healing by any form of the supernatural became impossible for science to take seriously. We propose that the way to reintroduce all that Descartes placed in abeyance as part of mind—which included the spiritual and hence the symbolic and cultural—with dualism is to reconceptualize and reformulate his thinking. Chapter 15 turns to science as a cultural process, concluding with some of the changes in thinking introduced by those attempting to transform the paradigm inherited from Descartes. Building on the innovative thinking of psychologist Ernest L. Rossi, the imagery of communication and information flow is outlined in chapter 16. Aspects of culture, such as the belief in what may cause and cure human suffering, viewed as information, may enter, as do suggestions made to an individual by a therapist, and flow, moving through the psyche to other bodily systems to the level of the molecules and cells. Beliefs about what spirits and other forms of the supernatural can accomplish may then turn on a specific category of genes to make amino acids that activate the endorphins, the body's own painkillers, or the immune system, contributing to the improvement of the patient and leading to recovery. In chapter 17, summarizing studies in hypnosis and successes achieved with hypnotically facilitated therapy, I propose, again following Rossi, that what anthropologists report as trance is comparable to hypnosis and that it is when a person is in such a state that the information content of suggestions—psychological or cultural—is most effectively transduced to turn on genes, molecules, cells, and bodily systems that aid in healing. The final chapter returns to the data presented in part I to show that the healing rituals of the diverse groups include a preliminary phase during which those who recover may enter an altered state of consciousness (ASC), during which the belief in spirits or other supernatural(s) stimulates bodily reactions leading to the cures reported. These are the people who convert. Those who do not enter an ASC and are not cured culturalbiologically are those who continue their quest in the religious marketplace.

My experience in Brazil would not have been possible without the cooperation and help of many people. I am indebted to the late Dr. Edson Queroiz, Dr. José Lacerda de Azevedo, and Antonio de Oliveira Rios for enabling me to observe and film their work. I wish to thank José Carlos Ribeiro, Mauricio Magalhães, Dr. Ivan Hervé, their coworkers, and all of the spirit guides; the mediums at the Casa de São Francisco and many other Kardecist centers; and the collaborators and patients at Spiritist centers who helped make the research possible. I wish to express my gratitude to the *pais- and mães-de-santo* at *terreiros* of Candomblé, Xangô, Batuque, and Umbanda throughout Brazil who have permitted me to observe and film their usually private rituals, especially my godson, the other José Carlos Ribeiro. I am grateful to the evangelical pastors, their parishioners, and the priests and monks at the monastery in Canindé and to the numerous pilgrims who shared with me their most personal experiences.

I am grateful to my friend and fellow anthropologist Dr. Antônio Mourão Cavalcante, professor and chair of the Department of Psychiatry at the Faculty of Medicine of the Federal University of Ceará and practicing psychiatrist, who welcomed us into his home as family, listened to my stories, and advised me on so many aspects of the research. It was he, along with Professor Adalberto Barreto, of the Faculty of Medicine at the Federal University of Ceará, who encouraged me to examine Spiritist healing and provided repeated opportunities for me to present some of the results at a series of conferences in Canindé.

Professor Roberto Motta of the Federal University of Pernambuco shared with me his extensive knowledge of Xangô and Afro-Brazilian religions and enabled me to gain access to many of the terreiros where I observed and filmed rituals. He participated significantly in much of what is reported in this volume.

Professor Cícero Marcos Teixeira, retired from the Faculty of Education of the Federal University of Rio Grande do Sul, has been an invaluable mentor and guide in Spiritism.

Sueli Schutz and her children, Paulo Andre and Karina, while coping with their own loss, welcomed my wife and me as if we were members of her family. Our enduring friendship is one of the unanticipated and cherished rewards of this work.

I am indebted to Professor Ari Pedro Oro of the Federal University of Rio Grande do Sul for all that I have learned from him about popular religions.

To Professor Luis Fernando Raposo Fontenelle, from whom I learned so much about Brazil during my many visits to Fortaleza and Rio de Janeiro, I am forever grateful.

Professor Conrad M. Arensberg, my teacher at Columbia University so many years ago, continues to influence my thinking.

It was Dr. Ernest L. Rossi from whom I learned psychobiology and hypnotically facilitated therapy. I thank him for his encouragement.

Robert Anderson, professor of anthropology at Mills College and an MD, accompanied me on visits to the Kardecist healer-mediums. I thank him for reading the manuscript and making valuable comments.

Fellow student of Spiritist healing Stanley Krippner, professor at the Saybrook Graduate School and Research Institute in California, taught me about hypnosis. I am grateful to him for reading the manuscript and helping improve it.

I remember the late Drs. Arnold Strickon and Morton Klass, classmates and colleagues with whom I discussed this research from its inception.

I wish to thank Jennifer Collier at Left Coast Press for her editorial suggestions and enthusiastic support. Immy Humes and Pablo Assunção helped to make the pictures that illustrate the text from my original videos. Artist Margo Magid caught the essence of the book in her creatively designed cover. I express my appreciation to the University Seminars at Columbia University for their help in publication. Some of the materials contained in this work were presented to the University Seminars on Brazil and Religion. This version has benefited from discussions in both seminars.

My wife, Eleanor, was my devoted companion on this adventure, as she has been in all aspects of my life for more than half a century. Without her support and encouragement, neither the research nor this report of it could have been accomplished. Our daughter Suzanne, a regular traveler to Brazil since her first birthday, and her brother David have contributed in more ways than I can ever adequately acknowledge. Our elder daughter, Jennifer, accompanied us many times and was in Fortaleza in 1981 conducting her own research. She shared in our excitement when we first met and observed José Carlos. I wish that Jennifer were still on this plane of reality to give me her professional judgment on how I have handled what she encouraged me to pursue. I alone accept responsibility for what is presented in the text.

Now we begin the journey into the world of religion, healing, and surgery by supernatural beings and into the efforts of an anthropologist to describe, analyze, comprehend, and explain the unusual phenomena I have been privileged to experience.

PART I

SURGERIES AND OTHER HEALING IN KARDECIST-SPIRITISM

CHAPTER 1
JOSÉ CARLOS RIBEIRO
AN INTRODUCTION TO SPIRITIST THERAPY

Anthropology demands the open-mindedness with which one must look and listen, record in astonishment and wonder at that which one would not have been able to guess.

Margaret Mead

The middle-aged man who had guided us through the mob on the street, into the big old house, and up a flight of stairs to a tiny bedroom, into which were crowded some two dozen people, pointed to a smiling, attractive, slender young man, probably in his late twenties, and announced, grinning broadly, "This is our healer." Like so many Brazilians, he was of mixed African and European descent. Wearing an open sport shirt and dark trousers, José Carlos Ribeiro needed only a guitar to look like an entertainer. Not the image I'd anticipated for a Spiritist healer who had already attained some notoriety in this bustling seaside city of Fortaleza on the north coast of Brazil. This man was reputed to do surgery without using any anesthesia or antisepsis.

After I was introduced and presented my wife, Eleanor, and teenage daughter, Suzanne, I told him that I was a scholar and researcher, adding a few sentences about my previous studies in Brazil and elsewhere.

My Portuguese was quite good, as I had been coming to Brazil for more than two decades to conduct research and teach. When I asked if we could observe him at work, José Carlos's smile faded momentarily.

"Do you work for a newspaper or magazine?"

"No. If I write anything, it will be for an academic or professional publication. I have no interest in sensationalism."

Apparently reassured, he smiled warmly. "I'll be delighted for you to watch. We have nothing to hide."

On the table he would later use for surgery there was a large tray with scalpels, several scissors, a few tweezers, a syringe, some cotton, gauze, adhesive tape, a glass of water, and a small pad of paper. He faced me again and placed the tray in my hands, adding, "Better than just watching, you can assist me."

Eleanor and Suzanne stared wide-eyed. I grasped the tray, realizing that my years of anthropological training and experience could not help to suppress my uncertainty and apprehension about what was to happen next.

José Carlos turned to a waiting patient, a simply dressed, dark-skinned, elderly man who was accompanied by his wife. As she started to explain her husband's vision problem, the healer shifted his eyes away from her toward the ceiling. Although I was unable to understand what he said next, I saw him begin to shake almost violently. Later, he told me that this happens when a spirit possesses his body.

Large numbers of Brazilians are convinced that spirits may take over the bodies of special individuals who are referred to as mediums. Initiates of African-derived religions, for example, enter trances, often while chanting or dancing, to embody supernatural beings believed to be from Africa or a mixture of African deities and Roman Catholic saints. Once possessed, they offer help with material as well as spiritual problems to fellow adherents or visitors.

But José Carlos was a follower of the Christian-oriented Kardecist tradition. Its conviction that spirits of the dead can communicate with the living has American and French origins (See Weisberg 2004; Greenfield 1987a; Cavalcanti 1983). Kardecist mediums become possessed without songs, dances, or sacrificial rituals. Being chosen by a spirit to serve as its medium often requires only the medium's own inner readiness; although, as we shall see, more often training programs are provided.

José Carlos interrupted the woman's account of her husband's symptoms: "Do you believe in God?" The soft tone of his previous speech was replaced by a sharp accent that sounded almost like a native speaker of Spanish trying to communicate in Portuguese. I did not yet know that the spirit believed to possess him was St. Ignatius of Loyola, the sixteenth-century founder of the Society of Jesus.[4] Before either of them could answer, he commanded: "Think of God! Think of God!"

Even as he issued this order, he picked up a scalpel from the tray I held and plunged it up under the lid of the upper rim of the man's left eye. Some of the onlookers gasped. One woman screamed. With a series of jabbing and twisting movements he slid the instrument down under the eye. Substituting the back of a tweezers taken from the tray with his left hand for the scalpel, he eased the eye forward, tilting it out of its socket. Using the scalpel still held in his right hand, he scraped what seemed to be the cornea of the protruding eye.

I was standing beside José Carlos, Suzanne behind me and Eleanor shoulder to shoulder with other onlookers behind the healer. I was struggling just to keep the tray in my hand from shaking or tilting. I allowed myself a momentary glance at my wife. Her face had turned pale, her mouth was hanging open, and her eyes were blinking rapidly. I feared she might faint. What could I do to help her? My mind seemed frozen.

José Carlos, without shifting his gaze from the old man in front of him, left the tweezers and eye dangling momentarily and moved his left hand over his shoulder. He barely touched Eleanor's face as he mumbled something I couldn't hear. Her complexion and expression almost instantly returned to normal. He once again gripped the tweezers.

He scraped the eye a few more times with the scalpel, then slid the tweezers to the top of the eye under the lid where the scalpel had first been thrust. He pulled the tweezers out. Back went the eyeball. All this happened in just a minute or two.

José Carlos covered the eye with some gauze and adhesive tape. "Did that hurt?" he asked. "Did you feel any pain?"

"No. I know what you did but I couldn't feel it."

The healer took a pen from his shirt pocket and the pad of paper from the tray and looked off into space as he wrote a prescription that seemingly flowed from the writing tool. He handed it to the old man's startled wife and rattled off a list of foods to be eaten or avoided, plus other orders about what her husband must and must not do.

"Go," he added, gesturing the couple away. "You will be well."

During the momentary pause between patients I looked at Eleanor. We both turned to our daughter: "You okay?"

She nodded, and with an uncertain smile, asked, "What have we gotten into?"

Still holding the tray, I shrugged, thinking about the happenstance that had brought us here. The previous morning I was relaxing on the balcony of our second-story apartment, enjoying the ocean breeze, browsing through the local newspaper, hearing the voices of my wife and daughters inside finishing their breakfasts. I wouldn't start teaching at the university until some weeks later.

I turned the page and changed my life.

The words "José Carlos Ribeiro" in a headline gripped my attention because that's the name of one of our Brazilian godsons. He had been born in our apartment in Rio de Janeiro during a research sojourn more than fifteen years previously. His mother was Maria, whom we had hired to assist Eleanor with toddler Suzanne and our two other children while I was off doing interviews and collecting data. After a few weeks with us, she had revealed her pregnancy. Months later we attended José Carlos's baptism, serving as his godparents in a rural village church.

"Ellie!" I shouted, almost as a reflex. "Look at this!"

She appeared on the balcony in moments, shadowed by slim, adolescent Suzanne. By then I had read the first paragraphs below the headline. Not our godson, but a Spiritist medium with the identical name. The coincidence seized my curiosity and led me to recall my reading about a man named Zé Arigó (see Fuller 1974), credited with doing spectacular surgeries without the use of anesthesia and antisepsis while in trance in the 1960s. The address where this José Carlos Ribeiro would be doing healing was in the paper.

"Let's see if we can meet him."

So early the next morning, we started our walk into downtown Fortaleza in search of this other José Carlos Ribeiro. Fortaleza, capital of the northeastern state of Ceará, is less than a hundred miles south of the equator. The temperature was already escalating. Still, we walked rapidly, both eager and anxious.

We turned a corner. Ahead of us, a couple hundred people stood in line in front of a large house, across from what we later learned were the offices of the National Health Services. Young and old, well to do and poor, a mix of racial identities—they were all seeking the healer I hoped to see in action.

The man facing the head of the line was ordinary looking, a typical northern Brazilian mixture of European and Indian. He was handing out numbers and tickets after a few words with each person. Trying to sound far more self-assured than I felt, I handed him my card identifying me as both an American professor and a visiting faculty member at the Federal University of Ceará's Department of Sociology and Anthropology for the semester beginning in August 1981.

"Would it be possible for me to meet the healer?" I asked.

He went to the doorway and talked with another gatekeeper. Then he motioned to us: "Come with me."

In a few minutes we were inside the house. No breezes reached the already steamy interior of the building. People crowded every available space. The murmur of their voices and odor of their bodies in the heat followed us up the flight of stairs to the room where we now stood.

Throughout the morning, the healer alternated between men and women, between those on whom he performed surgeries and those for whom he only wrote prescriptions. He removed cysts and tumors, repeated the popping out and scraping of eyeballs, and repaired what we thought was a detached retina. No one was given any anesthetic. The instruments on the tray were used repeatedly without being cleaned. In each case, diagnosis, surgery, bandaging, writing of a prescription for postoperative medication, and dictation of a list of behavioral restrictions and a special diet were all completed in a few minutes. Nonsurgery patients required even less time. José Carlos provided prescriptions for cures or to prepare patients for return visits and possible future surgeries.

Each time he wrote a prescription, he looked away from his hand and the pad of paper. Some of the medications were available at a regular pharmacy or in the market. Others could be found at an "Umbanda shop," where herbs, teas, baths, candles, and incenses are sold. A few were very obscure and difficult to obtain because they were so old in their formulations or so new that they were available only in the metropolitan centers of southern Brazil where the large, multinational drug companies had laboratories and outlets.

José Carlos, a high school graduate, had no further formal education. He did not charge fees for his consultations, diagnoses, prescriptions, surgeries, or other treatments. All were provided as charity. Brazilian Kardecist-Spiritists believe that healer-mediums receive spirits who in a previous lifetime were trained and practiced as doctors, surgeons, and other health care specialists. These spirits desire to perform the highly valued charitable act of helping the sick but do not need or wish to reincarnate (Greenfield 1987a).

Mediums possessed by such spirits provide various types of treatment. Passes may be administered, transmitting healing energy to the patient from the spirit world. Prescriptions are written, often for allopathic or homeopathic remedies. As we shall see, disobsessions—in which low-level spirits believed to be causing mental or physical illnesses are exorcised—are performed. Only a very small number of mediums perform surgeries.

José Carlos gave several patients prescriptions for a medicine obtainable only on the premises from his cousin or from a companion who travels with José Carlos as an assistant and confidant. Patients were charged the equivalent of four or five dollars to defray the cost of preparation, bottling, and shipping. Because of this payment, some in the Spiritist movement were to question José Carlos's integrity.

Late in the afternoon, the healer was approached by several people who came as a group on behalf of their brother, bedridden with a cancer diagnosed by his physician as terminal. Even as one of them was explaining why the stricken man was unable to come to this location, José Carlos was staring past them and writing a prescription.

"Give this to him. He can be cured. I will operate on him next week. But tomorrow morning I'll come see him."

It was evening before he finished with his last patient. Although the experience had left Eleanor, Suzanne, and me exhilarated but exhausted, he seemed full of energy. We'd been told that José Carlos would be back again in the morning.

"May I return and continue to observe your work?" I asked.

"Of course, of course." He smiled. "You were a fine assistant."

I laughed. After the fifth patient I had been relieved of my tray-holding duties.

Eleanor, Suzanne, and I headed for dinner and home in the warm night darkness. Our minds and conversation were whirlpools of questions without answers. How could we have seen what we saw? Who would ever believe us? Why had we not heard much more about Spiritist healers? How about casualties from the cutting without sterilizing instruments or using antiseptics on the wounds? Why would that large and very diverse crowd of patients choose to risk even prescriptions from this unlicensed and essentially untrained practitioner, to say nothing of being cut into by him without the slightest anesthesia? Were they somehow hypnotized? What about afterward? Had anyone ever checked to see if the people who submit themselves to this treatment actually get well? Or return for more treatments?

Our questions were very American. But the gentle breeze with its faint patina of garden perfumes reminded us that any answers would have to be Brazilian. This culture has elements from colonial Portugal, from the indigenous Indians whom the Portuguese conquered and impressed into plantation peonage, and from Africans imported as slaves. These elements have coalesced into a milieu that must be comprehended in its own terms.

We arrived the next morning as another crowd was gathering. Approaching the door at the same time were the brothers of the man José Carlos had promised to visit that day. They wanted to thank him for saving the man's life, invite him to lunch, and drive him and any assistants to where their brother lived.

"Last night," said the thin, intense one who did the talking the day before, "his whole body swelled up. We thought his veins would burst! Suddenly, he fell off his chair and we saw him bleeding. Our doctor came right away and told us to prepare for the end, probably before the night was over. He gave us a prescription for a shot of morphine to ease the pain and left. But we'd already gotten the medicine you prescribed just before the doctor came, and that's what we used."

The medicine had arrived by airline from Recife, capital of the neighboring state of Pernambuco, several hundred miles distant. This family of means and education, having searched Fortaleza's pharmacies in vain, prevailed on a friend with a ham radio to solicit help from contacts in other cities. It's difficult for most outside the Spiritist community to make sense of such effort and expense to carry out the instructions, not of a licensed, professional physician, but of an alleged healer with no training in modern biomedicine.

Adherents of Brazilian Spiritism, loosely organized by the Spiritist Federation, include practicing medical doctors, lawyers, university professors, engineers, architects, pharmacists, and other professionals who hold positions of prestige and importance in Brazilian society. Some are members of elite families who have traveled to and studied in North America and Europe. Many are well versed in Western, rationalist knowledge. Yet at times they choose to be operated on by healer-mediums lacking in medical training and credentials. Later we were to work with Spiritist healers even less educated than José Carlos.

As promised, José Carlos, his cousin, and several volunteer helpers arrived for an early lunch. The recipient of his prescription, apparently so close to death the night before, had already eaten but was still seated at the dining room table waiting to greet the healer. José Carlos sympathized with his patient's desire to walk to a nearby store to get a pack of cigarettes but sent him upstairs to his bedroom.

The healer ate the ample meal rapidly and engaged in good-humored conversation with family members and his own group. Afterward, he was accompanied upstairs by at least twenty onlookers. Once again he mumbled to himself, shook convulsively while looking at the ceiling, and spoke authoritatively with the same stilted accent: "I will operate on you next Thursday. Soon you will be well. Your cancer will be cured. Meanwhile, rest. Rest and take your medicine."

He turned from the bed and descended the stairs, once again talking in his normal voice.

We returned to the house full of people who had been waiting for his attention and treatment. José Carlos selected another "volunteer" assistant, a surgeon who was a friend and former classmate of the very patient just visited. A large man, middle-aged and with a precise mustache and an air of expertise, he had come to observe the practitioner into whose hands his friend's life had been placed.

They stood before an attractive young woman who was to be treated first this afternoon. Even before she spoke, José Carlos went through the process of entering trance. He then picked up a scalpel and drove it into her cheek so precisely that only a small incision was made. From this he drained a cyst and removed it in several pieces. She sat quietly for the brief time it took him, her oval face placid. After an assistant closed and bandaged the incision, she smiled a little.

The next few patients were given prescriptions. This break gave me a chance to ask the visiting surgeon, a licensed physician and not a Spiritist, about what I'd seen.

"In your professional opinion, how well was that done?"

"His technique was impressive," he replied. "Most physicians would have cut an incision four times that size in order to lift the cyst out whole. That is a less exacting technique but then it produces much more bleeding and surrounding tissue damage."

"Would it take less time that way? This happened pretty quickly."

He looked at me very directly: "I've never seen this done so quickly—a fraction of the time usually required."

"How could he have learned and perfected such skill?"

Poker-faced, the surgeon shrugged. I tried two more questions: "What about no anesthetic? And no antiseptic to clean the scalpel and the wound?"

Another shrug.

By a quarter after three, José Carlos was treating the last of the people who had gathered at this house to see him. Only then did I learn that he would be escorted immediately to another place, already teeming with others seeking his attention. After the second house, there would be a throng waiting for him at a third dwelling. He completed his work there by about five in the afternoon. We returned to the first house, where a jam-packed crowd had formed and was once again awaiting his return.

Without pausing to rest, he moved quickly from patient to patient—examining, diagnosing, writing prescriptions, dispensing his own medicine, performing more surgeries, and scheduling others. Well into the evening he saw the last patient here, but more awaited him at a suburban Spiritist center. That at last concluded the work for this second day. José Carlos glanced at a clock on the wall. It was almost ten at night.

"Dinner!" he exclaimed, looking at his assistants with a broad smile on a face that showed no sign of weariness. "We haven't had any dinner. We must eat!"

Six of us accompanied him to a beachfront restaurant that provided a singer along with delicious food. When the singer took a break, José Carlos moved to the microphone. He picked up the guitar left there and fulfilled my initial image of him as an entertainer, playing and singing to the obvious delight of the other patrons. I was able to hear the ocean drumming on the shore and retreating waves hissing about the sea's secrets. We ate, danced, and sang until after midnight.

At eight the next morning the healer was back at work, looking fresh and full of energy. After the night before, I felt well enough acquainted to use the pause for a hurried lunch to ask questions: How did he diagnose patients and decide what medicines to prescribe? Where did he acquire his surgical skills?

"I don't know how to answer you," he replied, "since I'm not the one who does this work." His tone was earnest, his expression without a trace of guile. "St. Ignatius does what is required for each of the patients. Afterward my assistants tell me what he had contributed through me to their well-being. I have no memory of the services rendered."

"How can you keep on working hour after hour into the night?" I asked, impressed with his energy and tenacity.

"Whenever I return from trance, I feel rested and relaxed, even at the end of the day."

On the fourth day, however, José Carlos appeared far from relaxed. He seemed agitated. When he was not in trance, there was an undertone of tension to his conversation, an uncharacteristic irritability. Once again, I used the brief lunchtime for conversation, wondering aloud if something was troubling him.

"They're after me." His youthful face was clouded with some mixture of anger and sadness. "The police received a complaint from the state medical society. I've been accused of violating the law prohibiting the practice of medicine without a license. They've warned me: Stop treating people and leave town or be arrested and charged."

"Can that actually happen?"

"Back in the early sixties, a well-known healer popularly known as Zé Arigó was put on trial, found guilty, and sent to jail. And he had far more well-placed supporters than I do."

"Why so much opposition to what you do?"

"Look across the street," he replied, referring to the offices of the National Health Services. "This is not a good place to have been rented for my work. Those doctors look out and see all these people waiting for treatments we give to them. Many must be covered by national health insurance—that would mean fees for those doctors if they didn't come here."

"Wouldn't they have known wherever you were located? After all, I read about you in the newspaper. And there's been mention on the radio."

For the first time José Carlos smiled a little. "Being under their noses may have been the last straw." He stood up, reached across the table, and put a friendly hand momentarily on my shoulder. "We must return to our patients."

Two days later, would-be patients arrived to find José Carlos gone. He'd retreated, unannounced, to a distant suburb, where he was still treating the few who knew of his move. But within days the media discovered and reported his activities. Again the long lines of those seeking his aid formed.

Maria Laura, the hostess of a local radio show on Spiritist themes, came to conduct an interview and observed the cousin collecting money for the special medicine. Without asking for an explanation, she denounced José Carlos on her program and in a newspaper column, accusing him of fraud. The issue had nothing to do with his treatments: there were no complaints, no reports of infections, deaths, or even worsened conditions. There was only the alleged violation of the Spiritist prohibition against receiving payments. But the accuser, daughter of European immigrants and owner of a dress factory, was an activist in the Spiritist community in Fortaleza. What she said carried weight.

Ten days after I first saw him, this healer with the same name as my godson quietly disappeared. The police were satisfied that they had done their job. The medical society was pleased to have protected the public. Those Spiritists opposed to him as a fraud for taking money rejoiced in the preservation of the purity of their beliefs. The cancer victim who anticipated the possibility of a miraculous surgery was in despair.

Two days earlier José Carlos had given me the address and telephone number for his home in Goiânia, capital of the interior state of Goiás. I tried the number from time to time over a period of two decades to no avail. In the future, on my way to see another healer in a nearby town, I went to the address. He was not there. I was neither to see nor hear of him again.

CHAPTER 2

EDSON QUEIROZ

SPIRITIST SURGERIES IN RECIFE

In 1983, in my hotel room in Recife, the capital of the northeastern state of Pernambuco, I watched a videotape of the next Spiritist healer-medium I was to meet: Edson Cavalcante de Queiroz. In his mid-thirties and wearing a physician's white jacket, he was assisted by a surgeon and a gynecologist. He asked them to examine the woman lying on an operating style table. She appeared to be in her fifties. Her left breast was exposed. Edson had already moved his fingers along its surface while gazing off into space. He told her there was a tumor, which he would remove. Stepping back, he gestured to the two assisting physicians.

"Please make your assessment." He had an accent although he was a native Brazilian.

As soon as they agreed with the healer's diagnosis, Edson commanded the woman, "Think of God. Pray! Think of God."

Even as he spoke, he took a scalpel and cut an inch-long incision into her breast. Although he hadn't washed his hands since treating the previous patient, he dug his fingers into the wound. They could be seen under the skin rapidly manipulating the tumor in the direction of the opening. The woman's lips were moving, although she made no sound. Her eyes were closed. A trickle of blood ran down the side of her breast.

Edson removed his fingers, retrieved his scalpel, and enlarged the opening a little. Reinserting his fingers, he slipped the tumor out. He handed it to the surgeon, who took it from the healer's ungloved, unwashed hand with a pair of tweezers and placed it in a sterilized jar to be sent to a laboratory for confirmation that it was benign.

"Come here," Edson commanded the surgeon and the gynecologist, indicating the place where he stood while operating. The woman continued to lie motionless on the table. "Take your dirty hands and put them inside her breast so that you may examine it. You will not infect her."

Each complied. Neither wore gloves. They concurred that the tumor had been removed.

Eighteen others in the room were witnessing the operations Edson performed that morning before television cameras in the city of Guaratingatá in the southeastern state of São Paulo. A crowd of more than two thousand had come to the Spiritist center to see him. He was a preeminent healer-medium and Spiritist surgeon, highly praised within the Spiritist Federation, even by Maria Laura in Fortaleza.

He was also a trained and licensed physician, a graduate of the medical school of the Federal University of Pernambuco. He practiced conventional medicine for fees at a private clinic specializing in gynecology and general surgery in Recife, where he lived with his wife and three children. Away from the clinic, whenever he provided free services as a medium-healer, he asserted that the work was done by the spirit of a Dr. Adolph Fritz, a German who was killed in 1914 while serving as head of a military hospital in the Kaiser's army.[5] Edson and his supporters founded the center in Recife where he did his surgeries in honor of Dr. Fritz.

After my experience with José Carlos in late 1981, I sought an introduction to Dr. Queiroz before leaving Brazil. On my way home I stopped in Recife, where we met at his clinic and discussed Spiritism and Spiritist healing. Warm, charming, open, and encouraging, Edson invited me to observe him at work whenever I returned to the city. An invitation to attend a conference there provided that opportunity and gave me a chance to continue researching Spiritist healing and surgeries. I already knew that this study had become the most compelling interest in my life.

Watching the video of Edson at work as a Spiritist healer, I tried to imagine him instead in the surgery room at his conventional clinic.

How do I reconcile the doctor and the medium being the same person? More important, how does he?

On the screen, a man slowly removing his jacket described the severe back problems that left him in constant pain. His wife had X-rays, taken by their personal physician, for Edson to review. He didn't even glance at them. Instead he asked the volunteer nurse assisting him for a scalpel.

"Think of God! Think of God!"

The scalpel was thrust through the man's shirt. I paused the picture. The blade was in deep enough to be scraping a vertebra, which is what Edson appeared to be doing vigorously when I resumed the playback.

"Needles, please."

The nurse handed him a closed package of ordinary, two-inch-long syringe needles. He stopped scraping, left the scalpel dangling, and jammed in two needles about an inch apart just below the incision. He slapped the man vigorously on both sides of his back and then thrust two more needles in at the left base of his spine.

Turning away from his patient, Edson picked up a needle used on a previous patient, jammed it into the stomach of the technician helping him, and jerked it out. Then he thrust a second used needle into the neck of the nearest observer and a third through the hand of another bystander. The face of each displayed real shock.

"Did I hurt you? Did I hurt you?" Edson asked with stifled laughter.

"No. No." They shook their heads, recovering from their surprise.

"I just wanted everyone to know that the needles don't hurt."

Didn't hurt! I exclaimed to myself. I knew damn well they would have hurt me.

Edson removed the dangling scalpel and needles from the man's back. "You'll be well."

What was this mature, adult, licensed physician doing, displaying a mysterious power as if he were a child or some primitive shaman? The duality is rooted in the history of Brazilian Spiritism.

As a belief system, modern Spiritism began in Hydesville, New York, in the mid-nineteenth century (Weisberg 2004; Moore 1977; Nelson 1969; Isaacs 1957). Recognition of the possibility of communication with the world of the spirits of the dead spread to other parts of North America and from there to Europe—first to Great Britain, where a vibrant movement developed, and then to France. In Lyon, schoolteacher Léon Dénizarth Hypolyte Rivail published the results of interviews he had conducted with enlightened spirits—through mediums—under the pseudonym of Allan Kardec (Kardec [1864] 1987, [1861] 1975, [1857] n.d.), thus first codifying the movement's beliefs. His first work, *The Spirits' Book*, was published in 1857, followed by *The Medium's Book* in 1861. Copies of these seminal works were brought to Brazil, where they were first read in the original French by the elite and later translated for the masses (Bastide 1978; Renshaw 1969).

The number of followers of Kardec, though never large, grew, as did his influence in the development of Brazil's popular religions. Kardec saw his efforts as a reinterpretation of Christianity, which he believed had gone astray. He taught that in the beginning, God created not one world but two. We are part of the material world. The second, inhabited by spirits, remains unknown to us except for communication between spirits in that domain and the few on our plane gifted as mediums. According to Kardec, the spirits are the vital force in this dual universe. They animate both planes of reality. Morally driven toward progress, they return to the material world periodically to be presented with lessons, which, if learned, will move them along their path toward (spiritual) perfection, after which they will no longer have to reincarnate. Having free will, a spirit may choose to live out a life and disincarnate, returning to the spiritual plane without mastering the lesson, but then it will have to come back to repeat the same lesson at another time until it is learned.

Occasionally such a spirit was a healer in a previous earthly life, perhaps a physician. In that case, in a practice that appeared first in Brazil, it may use another mortal to accomplish healing as charity on our plane of reality.

Spiritists define morality in Judeo-Christian terms and acknowledge Jesus Christ as the most advanced spirit ever to have incarnated on the planet. His life is seen as the exemplar of moral perfection. His words, especially as set forth in the Gospels, as Kardec ([1864] 1987) interpreted them, are taken as expressing all that is virtuous.

At the heart of the Kardecist view of goodness in the world is charity. "Without charity," wrote the codifier (and his followers assert), "there is no salvation." Spiritist beliefs have come to be referred to as the ethic of practical charity (Renshaw 1969:74). "Spiritism without charity is inconceivable: It just is not Spiritism" (St. Clair 1971:115).

Spiritist charity took two main forms in Brazil: the giving of social assistance to the poor and healing (McGregor 1967:93). As each spirit goes through its individual trajectory, incarnating in the material world, disincarnating and reincarnating again across the millennia, while not always consciously aware of the moral imperative to do good and avoid evil, from the decisions and choices it makes it accumulates what some Brazilian Spiritists refer to as its karma: the moral balance of all of its previous experiences and choices.

Dr. Edson Queiroz's and his fellow Spiritists' beliefs do not lie much outside the mainstream sense of a spiritual dimension to life that pervades Brazilian culture. And how far is it, I reflect, from the sense shared by so many in my own country that miraculous cures have been performed by saints and that angels are quite real, visible or not?

I watched the video several more times, looking for clues to some alternative explanation, speculating about mass hypnosis. When I arrived at the Spiritist Federation headquarters the next day, volunteers in charge of protecting the healer from reporters seeking to sensationalize his activities stopped me. Apparently unaware of our plan to meet, they refused to tell him I was there, but Edson spied me from across the room. He came over and greeted me with a traditional Brazilian embrace, our arms around each other's shoulders, hands firmly patting.

"Welcome! Welcome!"

He smiled broadly. His somewhat round face, framed by a fashionable haircut with neatly trimmed mustache and short beard, was both animated and relaxed. He still had one arm around my shoulders as he introduced me to those by whom I had been intercepted. After that I was given carte blanche to roam the premises.

"Tomorrow, starting at seven in the morning, I will see my patients," he told me. "Make your preparations to watch and film my work."

Early morning sunshine highlighted the faces of the people patiently standing in long lines outside the federation's building—men and women, youthful and elderly, many chatting with those next to them, some quiet, others withdrawn. They all hoped to see the healer that day, but most would have to return for treatment in the days to come.

One volunteer gave out numbers. Another handed out cards, requesting that each would-be patient write a brief biography, a short statement of the symptoms or problem, any diagnosis from a previous doctor or healer, and the name of that practitioner. Other volunteers filled out cards for those who were unable to write. The twenty men and women Edson saw that morning included rich and poor, educated and illiterate, with various skin colors. Three were themselves practicing physicians, and one was a medical student.

A distinguished-looking middle-aged man, who I later learned was a practicing orthodontist, approached me. He was the president of the Spiritist Federation.

"We're about to start," he said.

We entered the building and went into a small alcove where a dozen people sat on a circle of chairs. I was introduced to officers from Spiritist groups in other states who had come to observe. The president began to read from a Spiritist version of the Gospel. After fifteen minutes Edson entered and quietly took a seat. As the reading continued, he changed visibly. His body quivered, his eyes bulged, his face was fixed in a stern expression—it was the appearance of the persona of Dr. Adolph Fritz. He took over the prayer session, speaking in a higher tone than I'd heard before, with what seemed to be a German-like accent and a strong sense of authority.

"All is ready now," he announced. He walked from the alcove. Even his gait had changed.

The sparsely furnished space provided for him was arranged like a doctor's clinic. A large inner room was curtained off to serve as a waiting area and an office. Here a doctor sat, prepared to write prescriptions and instructions dictated by Edson. Beyond her desk, two other doctors would assist the healer in his examinations. As I set up my equipment, he ordered the first patient to be brought in. He glanced through a pile of cards placed on the desk for him.

The hours that followed provided a veritable anthology of Spiritist surgeries.[6] Seeing them through the viewfinder of my video camera reminded me of the tape I had watched two nights before. The first two reprised the removal of a tumor from a woman's breast and the

(Upper left) Edson Querioz/Dr. Fritz inserting unwashed fingers into incision made in patient's throat after removing tumor. (Upper right) Edson Querioz/Dr. Fritz inserting unwashed fingers into incision made in patient's shoulder to remove growth. (Mid left) Edson Queiroz/Dr. Fritz inserting needles in patient's throat. (Mid right) Edson Queiroz/Dr. Fritz inserting needles in patient's back. (Lower left) Edson Queiroz/Dr. Fritz performing eye surgery. (Lower right) Edson Queroiz incorporating Dr. Fritz.

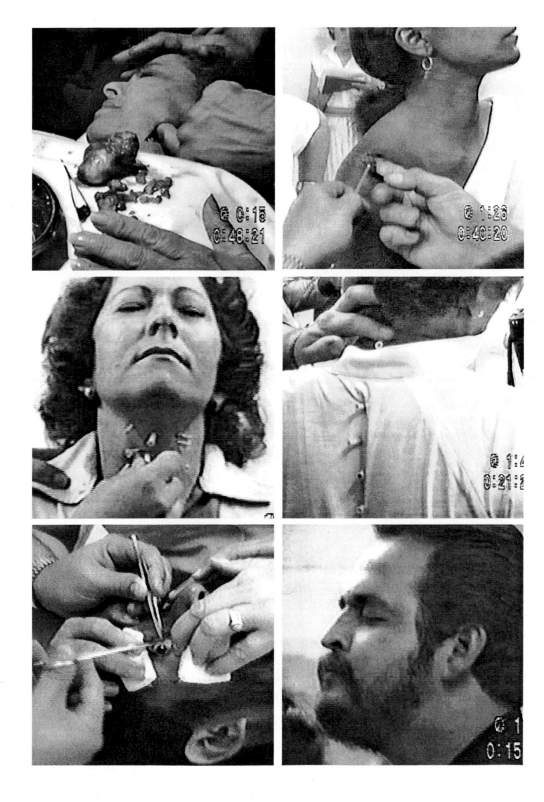

scraping of a scalpel against an upper vertebra—this time of an army captain, also with chronic, severe back pain.

The third patient was a diplomat who was almost blind in his right eye and now had the vision in his left blurred by a growth. He was accompanied by his brother, a professor at a university in the south of Brazil. After a cursory examination, Edson told him to lie on the makeshift operating table. Among those standing in the now crowded room was a local eye surgeon.

"Would you assist me with this?" Edson asked him. Given the Teutonic accent and authoritativeness of Dr. Fritz, the request was almost a command. After a moment's hesitation, the eye surgeon came to the healer's side.

"You can see what we have.[7] Have you removed such a growth in your practice?"

"Yes. Of course."

"How long does it usually take?"

"Thirty minutes or so."

"Who has a stopwatch?" Edson asked those in the room. Several men raised their hands, thereby displaying the large, multifunction gold wristwatches favored by many Brazilian professionals. The healer's own smaller gold wristwatch and band gleamed on his left wrist. He wore it throughout his operations.

"Time this," Edson said as he picked up a pair of scissors with his already bloodstained right hand and turned to the diplomat lying on the table. "Think of God. Do not move your eye. Think of God!"

He secured the end of the growth with tweezers in his left hand, snipped at the film, and pulled it free. "How long? How long?"

"Twenty-five seconds!" exclaimed one of those with stopwatches. The others concurred.

Edson turned to the eye surgeon: "Try to match that next time." Obviously, the spirit of Dr. Fritz didn't value modesty, but what came next was far more startling.

Turning to one of his regular assistants, he ordered him to spit in the open eye before a nurse covered it with gauze and a bandage.

"There will be no infection." That statement began a short sermon on how much conventional medicine still had to learn. "I don't oppose it. But the doctors of the medical establishment are closed-minded. They could learn much to benefit their patients if they would study what I do instead of bringing legal charges against me."

At the moment, I was too engrossed by what was happening to think about the issue Edson had raised. But it returned to my mind again and again, regarding not only the medical profession in Brazil but in the United States as well.

While Edson spoke, the diplomat sat up and drank the treated water given to each patient. As his brother assisted him toward the door, the healer asked how he felt. "Quite all right" was the reply.

I followed after with a few questions of my own and learned that the patient had been aware of all that had happened and had felt no pain. I was not surprised. It was what José Carlos's patients had told me. I would hear it from most of Edson's and those of healer-mediums I would meet later.

An overwhelming fear of pain brought the next patient, a young woman, to Edson. Fatima had refused to allow a conventional doctor to remove a growth from her right shoulder, even with the promised use of local anesthesia. She came with her mother, who had heard stories of Edson's operations without pain.

"Sit here," the healer said, pointing to a small operating table with his left hand. He held his right hand out to the professional nurse assisting him, who handed him a new scalpel still in its sterile container.

Fatima sat motionless, her oval face placid as he snapped the wrapping off the scalpel. He thrust it into her shoulder. Her expression remained unchanged—she made no sound, no movement. The nurse used a piece of gauze to pat the little trickle of blood oozing from the base of the cut and it stopped. Edson traded his scalpel for a scissors. He jabbed it into the open wound, pulled with it at the growth, and finally pushed his fingers into the red-lined opening to tear the infected material loose. Since he hadn't washed his hands after the previous operations, the sterility of the scalpel was patently irrelevant.

Fatima didn't flinch during the minute or so this took. The healer handed the growth to his pathologist, who would prepare a report, then placed a piece of adhesive over the open wound.

"We don't need to suture this," he said to the young woman and her mother standing at her side. Fatima offered a slight smile as the nurse bandaged over the adhesive and then directed them to the other side of the room to receive the glass of treated water. In the few moments this took, Edson wrote a prescription. Like José Carlos, he looked neither at his hand nor the paper. Here, too, the words appeared as if flowing from the pen.

Ready for his next patient, he was working at a pace that compelled my intense and continuous attention. But a thought I'd had before flashed through my mind as I squinted into the camcorder's viewfinder: Can any of this be trickery?

I was aware of a group in the United States called the Committee for the Scientific Investigation of Claims of the Paranormal (CSICOP).[8] James Randi, the group's leading spokesperson, had his own foundation dedicated to debunking a range of behaviors, including forms of healing that he considered fraudulent. He and his colleagues used the most sophisticated techniques of professional magicians to reproduce events that even a few scientists thought lay beyond the explanations of natural science. In Randi's 1982 book, a chapter called "The Medical Humbugs," based on filmed scenes of Zé Arigó, dismissed the surgeries as especially clever illusions. He compared that famous Spiritist with the much-publicized Philippine "psychic surgeons," who did not really cut but often pretended to do so, slipping vials of animal blood and tissue into their clothing and then showing them as if they came from the patient (Randi 1982). In a 2005 episode of ABC's *Primetime Live,* and in a written critique following the program, Randi debunked the work of João Teixeira de Farias, another Spiritist healer-medium known by English speakers as John of God (see Randi 2005; ABC 2005). He further asserted that academics and scientists were especially susceptible to being taken in by such superb frauds.

Was I being taken in? If so, then my company included not only hundreds of Spiritist patients but also other professional medical providers—doctors and nurses—who assisted Edson regularly or as volunteers chosen at one or another moment. This group included the licensed pathologist who was called upon again in the treatment of the next patient.[9]

The patient was middle-aged. Her dress and demeanor suggested low social status and little means. She could scarcely walk but had struggled to the Spiritist center on crutches, assisted by relatives. Told like the others to think of God, she sat quietly on the operating table as Edson forcefully jabbed syringe needles into her back just two or three inches apart in a descending line along her spinal column. He inserted the last needle just above the base of the spine.

"A test tube," he commanded the assisting pathologist. In it he collected what he said, and the pathologist agreed, was spinal fluid that had started to flow. When the tube was a third full, he handed it back.

"A complete analysis," he ordered.

Then he slapped the woman's back quite forcefully and rapidly removed the needles. She was still startled as he said, "You will be fine."

Magic?

Another woman, suffering from sinus problems and a chronically stuffed nose, was seated on an examining chair, her head tilted back. Edson drove a pair of scissors up into her left nostril, deep into the sinus cavity. Then he wrapped a second pair with gauze, asked a bystander to spit on it, and jammed it up into the other nostril.

"No infection," he said once again. "No infection."

Fakery? Suppose all of us were somehow being deceived by legerdemain. Yet how could even the most adroit sleight of hand accomplish antisepsis? I had to come more directly to grips with the "Amazing" Randi's assertions. When I returned home, I studied the magician's craft, especially tricks that give the illusion of cutting and surgery. My instructor also arranged for me to show videotapes of the surgeries I'd witnessed to almost four hundred practicing magicians at a magician's convention in Chicago. They concurred that this wasn't stagecraft or sleight of hand. The healer was really cutting and jabbing into his patients, who were bleeding from actual wounds.

Edson's last patient before lunch that day was himself a physician. He had his own clinic in Copacabana, an elite section of Rio de Janiero. Distinguished looking, probably in his sixties, he was dressed in a well-tailored three-piece suit. Above its collar protruded a large bandage on the left side of his neck. Edson removed the bandage, exposing an infected, festering growth. I imagined that up close it must smell. One of the assisting physicians muttered aloud the question that came to my mind and no doubt occurred to many other observers: "How could a doctor let something like this go on so long without treatment?"

Edson disregarded the remark with its implications of both bewilderment and dismay. "Take off your jacket and tie. Loosen your shirt. Lie down here." He pointed to the operating table. "On your side."

He clamped onto the mass with a pair of forceps and jabbed into it with a scalpel, pulling upward even as he cut. Blood spurted out, more than we'd seen so far that morning. He put down the scalpel and took from the nurse pieces of gauze, which he placed over the wound. He looked over at those of us who were watching.

"I permit this much bleeding this time so you can see that it comes from the wound, that this is not a trick. No blood from chickens, like those Philippine psychic healers use."

I dismissed the thought that he was reading my mind as foolish. The bleeding quickly subsided, and Edson again sliced into the infected area, pausing only to control further bleeding. When about half the growth had been cut away, he put down his scalpel and again looked at us.

"Ask your questions," he said.

We'd been so absorbed in the operation that at first only silence greeted his invitation. Then several voiced their concerns. To each he responded with a mini-lecture on Spiritism. Meanwhile, his patient, like all who had preceded him, lay quiet on the operating table, eyes half closed in an obviously relaxed face.

Edson returned with renewed vigor to carving away the infected, discolored flesh. Another two minutes and the growth was completely removed, leaving a raw indentation that was covered with gauze for the moment to stop the bleeding. Then the healer spread an ointment over the shining wound, commenting, "This really isn't necessary. But patients feel better if I do it. And so will most of you watching this, to say nothing of members of the medical profession."

The attending pathologist received the removed tissue for laboratory analysis. The man sat up, and his wound was bandaged.

"You may go," Edson said in a friendly manner. "Remove the bandage in a few days. It will heal without a scar."

I followed the man toward the door. "Excuse me," I said, "but may I ask you something?" I quickly explained who I was and what I was doing. "Can you tell me what you experienced during your operation?"

"I could feel the cutting, but without any pain." His voice was soft, dignified. "I feel fine, now, and I'm relieved that's finally done."

"You are yourself a doctor. When the growth first appeared, why didn't you go to one of the surgeons in Rio? Why come to Edson?"

He held himself especially straight and looked at me very directly as he responded: "I wanted to get at the *source* of the problem. Conventional doctors only treat symptoms and work at the surface. If you want to get at the cause, you go to a Spiritist healer-medium. Edson is the best. So I had to wait until I could come to Recife for his services."

Clearly, he was himself a follower of Spiritist doctrine. His conviction and sincerity were compelling. Yet in spite of all I'd seen, heard, and read up to that point, I didn't feel that I really understood what he meant by "getting at the source."

When I returned to Brazil the following year, I visited the doctor at his penthouse on Avenida Atlántica overlooking Rio's Copacabana Beach. He looked very well. "Yes," he assured me, "my health is excellent." He was wearing a sport shirt that fully revealed his neck. There was no trace of a scar.

As the elevator took me down to the sun-drenched street, I continued my struggle to understand what I'd seen of Spiritist surgeries, confronting my own contending beliefs, images, and feelings. Ways of thought developed to pursue my work as a cultural anthropologist are now almost second nature to me. I seek to "get inside" the culture I'm trying to understand—to hear its sounds, appreciate the power of its beliefs, know its tastes and odors, move along the pathways that bring order to experience, comprehend its sense of what is real. That's what I'd done through many immersions into Brazilian life, and that of the British Caribbean where I had worked previously. But followers of Kardecist-Spiritism share a special version of that culture. And I'm still also a creature of my own upbringing in an American society permeated by faith in Western technology and science, with its convictions about what constitutes evidence and proof.

At least performance magic had been ruled out. Some sort of hypnotic suggestion could have been part of what was going on. The followers of Spiritism considered their own doctrine as sufficient explanation. Yet many of them were receptive to my efforts to explore the matter further.

But how? The medical mainstream, even in medical anthropology, explains successful healers within a frame of reference that constrains analysis to so-called psychosomatic illnesses. Physical diseases and injuries are excluded almost by definition. For such ailments, only modern biomedicine offers "real" cures.

I was no longer able to accept this simplistic distinction as I walked away from a physician who had undergone a relatively painless removal of a large, deeply embedded growth without antisepsis or anesthesia because, in his own words, he wanted to get at the source and obtain a "real" cure. Most of the Spiritist surgeries I'd seen thus far had dealt with physical ailments and injuries. For that matter, what could be more physical than the operations I'd witnessed? Prevailing distinctions between mind and body blurred for me. Reality itself verged on the surreal.

In the United States, there have always been people who report cures and healing elsewhere than in hospitals and doctors' offices. Crutches are abandoned at religious shrines. Ministers lay on hands in the tradition of New Testament text. Jewish mystics provide curative blessings. For some of my countrymen, guardian angels are not mere metaphors but are almost palpable. However, most of those with whom I grew up and went to school disregarded reports of such experiences or considered them delusional, as do most of my professional contemporaries.

I smiled at the irony as I walked along the palm-lined boulevard with the ocean surf singing of eternities over the sounds of traffic. I could have found people involved in types of spiritualist healings in New York City, in Miami, in Appalachia, in the desert country of the Southwest, and of course all over California. But only here in Brazil could I find so physical, so observable a manifestation of what modern biomedicine can neither explain nor honestly dismiss.

A thin thread of history wound from the United States to Allan Kardec in France and then to Brazil. After the Fox sisters (see Weisberg 2004), in the 1840s attempts to contact the spirits of the dead became popular in North America. Sweeping across the United States, the practice crossed the Atlantic, spreading séances through England and onto the Continent. By the late nineteenth century, Ouija boards and table turning were common diversions for the upper classes in Brazil as well as in the United States, England, and France. Kardec stopped writing academic textbooks and undertook codifying Spiritist beliefs and practices. In two of the previously mentioned volumes, he published the answers to more than a thousand questions that, he asserted, he had asked of "enlightened spirits" with whom he had communicated through a pair of mediums.

Brazil, with its confluence of European, Indian, and African cultures, provided fertile soil for these ideas to take root and flourish. The powerful patron-dependent tradition, rooted in the Catholicism that the Portuguese brought to this country, was and is conducive to the relationship between spirits and those who seek their guidance. By the turn of the twentieth century, a Spiritist Federation was functioning here.

As I hailed a taxi I decided that, for the time being, I would not try to resolve the contending explanations and competing voices. Most immediately, I had to prepare for my next encounter with a Spiritist healer-medium.

CHAPTER 3

ANTONIO DE OLIVEIRA RIOS IN PALMELO

Some of the surgeries by Brazilian Spiritist healers that I had witnessed and videotaped were similar to treatments provided by conventional medical doctors. Growths inside and outside the body were removed and pterygiums scraped from eyes. But more treatments were performed only to "let the spirits in to do their work," as the healers repeatedly told me. Other than the fact that no healing was expected to ensue from the cutting that simulated actual (arthroscopic) surgery, how did this process differ from the so-called placebo surgeries performed on the arthritic knees and other organs of patients in the United States by licensed physicians in conventional hospital settings? It was not uncommon for those receiving this invasive placebo to do as well or better than the patients receiving "actual" treatment.

Inquiries exploring the contention that placebos often are not medically neutral but serve to activate healing processes in the patients receiving them are underway. Sometimes the differences between the effects of the placebos and the designated treatments (most often drugs) are very small, and the placebos have no destructive side effects.

I'm forced to ask myself: Might some of the work of Spiritist surgeons have such positive placebo effects? Like conventional medically approved surgeries, they are physical assaults on the bodies of patients, a kind of benign violence. Is this a contradiction in terms or a commonplace reality that we often ignore for ideological reasons?

The small, rural town of Palmelo in the state of Goiás, about sixty miles from the national capital Brasília, provided a striking contrast to the cosmopolitan urban centers of Fortaleza and Recife. The Spiritist healer-medium here, Antonio de Oliveira Rios, was an equally far cry from Dr. Edson Quieroz. There was no entourage of nurses and assistants to help him. A white jacket covered his broad shoulders. He wore rubber gloves and a surgical mask over his short, jet-black beard. The healer selected a scalpel from among two dozen tarnished, unsterilized instruments on a wheeled cart. Scissors, clamps, scalpels, and pads of gauze lay in disarray on a white towel. A large red stain bloomed at one end.

Shirtless, a stocky young man with dark hair lay prone on a gurney next to the cart. We were outside the Templo Espírita Dr. Ricardo Dwannees Stan, which housed Antonio's little clinic. The bright Sunday afternoon sun sharpened a shadow cast across the healer and his patient by an extension of the center's roof slung across the walkway alongside the small white building. Victim of a bullet wound ten years before, this man was still unable to use his legs. He came to see Antonio from the burgeoning metropolitan center of São Paulo.

A sweetness from nearby gardens mixed in the still air with the acrid odor of dust from the dirt road running to the center of the town. A large crowd stood restlessly in the heat looking on. Their murmuring mingled with the cheerful beats of recorded Latin rock music. Some were waiting for treatment. Others were only curious. Dressed casually, I could have been a waiting patient, except that I stood near Antonio holding a camcorder.

All watched intently as Antonio sliced into his patient. From the middle of the bare back to a few inches below the neck, the scalpel cut upward about half an inch deep alongside the patient's spinal column. Flesh pulled apart; a rivulet of blood flowed from the base of the cut. The man was conscious. Like the others, he had been given no anesthesia.

Antonio patted at the blood with some gauze and then placed two pads to soak up the continuing flow. He sliced along the wet red groove several more times. His left hand dabbed with a swab that he left lying at the bottom end of the glistening gash. He picked up a scissors and jammed it into the gaping wound, angled toward the spine. With another scissors he hammered on it, driving it deeper. The closest bystanders heard steel "thunk" against bone. Antonio paused briefly, repeated the procedure, pulled out the scissors, and dropped it on the cart. His patient made no sound or movement.

Antonio was a bricklayer by trade. He was semiliterate, having only a first-grade education. He had not read even the shorter, simpler writings published by contemporary Brazilian Kardecist-Spiritists. But when he worked as a healer, he and his patients believed that the spirit of Dr. Ricardo Stams, a German who had been trained in Italy a century before, possessed him.

No school of medicine ever taught his next action. Onlookers pushed closer as the healer-medium bent over and took from the lower shelf of the cart an electric saw with a serrated circular blade, four inches in diameter. An extension cord was handed to him through an open window at the side of the building. He plugged in the tool.

Antonio returned to his motionless patient, turned on the saw, and inserted its spinning blade at the base of the open wound. A carpenter of the flesh, he noisily enlarged the split in skin and muscle alongside the spinal column. Blood spurted up. The roadside chorus of onlookers gasped and muttered. The young man from São Paulo remained absolutely still, as if indeed only a board.

Finished cutting, Antonio turned off the saw, disconnected it, removed the blade, and returned the parts to the cart. Without so much as a glance at his handiwork, he hurried the cart with the tools through the door into the building where his next patient waited. The previous patient lay quietly on the gurney, unattended, still oozing a little of the red sap of life.

After a few minutes, a seamstress replaced the carpenter. Antonio's wife, a buxom woman with blond hair, also wearing a white jacket, came briskly out of the building with a large needle in one hand and surgical thread in the other. She quickly sutured up the slash in the man's back, covered the area with a bandage secured with tape, and immediately strode back into the center. Three friends who had helped him travel from São Paulo to Palmelo assisted the patient in sitting up. Onlookers converged with questions.

"How did it feel? Did it hurt? Did it hurt?"

He answered them as he was eased off the gurney back into his wheelchair. "No. No pain. Well, with the saw ... that was a little uncomfortable."

His friends helped him into the backseat of a car parked nearby. They drove off.

A little uncomfortable? I had an impulse to laugh out loud at the sheer incongruity between what this man had just experienced physically and what he must have felt—or didn't feel. As I waited for the next operation, I wondered if the issue of pain would provide an opening through which the mystery of Spiritist surgeries could be penetrated. Had Antonio's patient been injected with a local anesthetic, it wouldn't have been surprising that he remained conscious but felt little pain. Spiritist surgeons somehow seem to accomplish what anesthesiologists do with drugs and chemicals.

Unfortunately, medical science cannot as yet tell exactly what that is, even though a century and a half has passed since a physician from Georgia first tried ether. Anesthesiology has developed primarily by experimentation. Scientific methods have refined the craft but have failed to provide a secure theory for what it does. The various explanations, individually and taken together, remain incomplete. Perhaps transmission is decreased across neural synapses, the gaps between nerve cells. Or perhaps energy produced within cells to generate impulses is diminished, or nerve-impulse conduction is interfered with within cells.

Obviously, something prior to Antonio's first slice with a scalpel affected the nervous system of the man on the gurney at the level of molecules and electron flows required to produce anesthesia. It happened although neither Antonio nor his patient knew anything about neurotransmitters, much less which ones might prevent nerve cells from sending the brain information that would be experienced as pain. And it happened without anything being inhaled or injected.

I know that people other than Spiritist practitioners accomplish this. In China acupuncture is used to produce anesthesia for surgeries more profound than anything done by José Carlos, Edson, or Antonio. Advanced practitioners of yoga can control their own experiences of pain, as well as blood flow and bleeding. Some who suffer from migraine headaches have had success with biofeedback. Anesthesia for surgeries has been induced through hypnosis. A number of the professional magicians at the Chicago convention where

I showed videotapes of the surgeries pointed out signs that patients were in a state resembling what magicians try to evoke among members of an audience.

What is so puzzling, then, is not that (local) anesthesia is accomplished without the use of anesthetics, but that it occurs seemingly without the healers or their patients doing anything they are aware of to intentionally change what is happening at the level of synapses, receptors, and the generation, flow, and blocking of the most subtle energies—that is, unless I'd failed to see something because I did not know what to look for. Just as I'd studied magic, I had to learn about hypnosis and hypnotherapy.

I focused my camcorder's viewfinder on another patient still on a gurney in the shade at the side of the Spiritist center. In contrast with Antonio, he was an educated and sophisticated businessman who had flown to Palmelo from São Paulo. He was on his back with his shirt off. Antonio reappeared with his cart of instruments and pads. Blood from previous work had been wiped from the cutlery with a frayed, stained towel. His gloves and jacket, open at the collar like a sport shirt, were unchanged. Quickly he picked up a scalpel.

Before the healer could make his first cut, the man said something. Although those closest strained to hear, they couldn't quite discern what the ensuing, intense conversation was about. Still chatting, Antonio suddenly stabbed the scalpel into the right side of the man's abdomen about two inches above his black, belted blue pants. I had not seen nor caught on tape anything that I could imagine might have induced a trance, much less anesthesia.

With a continuous motion, the healer sliced up and leftward to just below the front arch of the rib cage. Aided by a scissors in his other hand, he swiftly cut the bloody, eight-inch gash deeper. He spread its edges apart to more than an inch and a half separation at the lower end. He jabbed his two instruments into the wound and moved them around. When he withdrew them, they brought along a small strip of shiny flesh. This, he told me later, was to better enable the spirits to deal with his patient's heart and arteries. The excised tissue was dropped into a jar containing a clear liquid.

Five separate red rivulets ran down the man's side. Where the skin had been peeled back, the slick, wet surface of underlying flesh and muscle was revealed. Blood bubbled out vigorously at the base of the cut, as if a small artery might have been snipped. The man on the gurney, seemingly oblivious to what his body was experiencing, continued his conversation with Antonio, who laid one of his scissors on the upper left side of the patient's chest and the other, along with the scalpel, on his stomach just above his belt. A fly buzzed by next to the Spiritist surgeon, looped around once, and flitted off.

Antonio dabbed a surgical gauze pad into the eight-inch-long wellspring for the little streams of blood flowing down the man's side onto the white pad under him. The flow slowed, almost stopped. After a few moments more of conversation, Antonio placed another gauze pad into the base of the wound where the cut was widest and bloodiest, then walked back into the building.

Alone now, the man on the gurney raised his head up and looked down across his chest at the healer's handiwork. His face displayed no sign of pain or concern. He lowered his head back onto the pad and closed his eyes, as if relaxing into a nap.

In a few minutes Antonio's wife once again appeared with needle, surgical thread, and bandages. A little blood still seeped from the wound as she stitched the edges together. The patient opened his eyes and began to chat with her as he had with her husband. When she was satisfied with her stitchery, she covered the sutured area with gauze and adhesive tape.

"Stand up, please," she told him, then helped him sit, turn sideways on the gurney, and slide off onto his feet. Many in the crowd were patently startled by what they were seeing. She wrapped his stomach and lower chest with a wide bandage, the outer end secured with tape.

"Now you can put your shirt on." She helped him slip his arms into it and left.

I had stopped videotaping. Perhaps my face, no longer hidden by the camcorder, revealed the anxiety I may have been feeling, even though I had seen such operations before. The patient smiled at me as he buttoned his shirt.

"I'm quite comfortable," he said as if to reassure me. "The same as when Antonio first operated on me."

He already knew that I was an American anthropologist and that I had been videotaping the operations that day as part of my research.

I nodded my head. "All this remains hard for me to understand."

His smile widened. "Perhaps that's because it's hard for you to believe."

He took a business card from his wallet and handed it to me. "Please, if you come to São Paulo, look me up and see how I'm doing."

I didn't have to wait that long. The next day at the nearest commercial airport— in Goiânia, a two-hour jeep ride from Palmelo—I saw him again. We were both waiting for our flights. He introduced me to his brother, who had accompanied him to help as needed. They looked a good deal alike, both square faced with trim mustaches, although Antonio's patient was clearly the older.

"You couldn't know it," the younger one said to me, "but a surgeon operated on my brother not long ago and told him it was hopeless. His arteries were so stuffed there wasn't much they could do. They gave him six months to live—at the most!"

"That's when we decided to try Antonio again," added the man whose chest I'd seen sliced and scissored. "Now I have something to show my doctor back in São Paulo," he continued with some excitement, reaching into his carry-on bag. He took out the small jar containing the tissue Antonio had removed from his chest.

After a little more conversation, my flight was called. We shook hands and wished each other well. Speaking to the younger brother by phone several times over the next two and a half years, I learned that the man with impacted arteries survived. He did well, traveling and not noticing any more symptoms of heart trouble.

I gazed out the window at the familiar Brazilian landscape below, thinking again about anesthesia without any anesthetic. Could there have been some connection between the history of hypnotism and the development of Kardecist-Spiritism? In the late eighteenth century, the Austrian physician Franz Anton Mesmer developed a theory he called animal magnetism as an alternative to then-accepted explanations of illness (see Fuller 1982; Mesmer 1980). In his practice in Paris, he claimed to use magnetism to induce healing. For that treatment, he brought his patients into a trancelike state by placing them "in a tub, a *baquet,* out of which magnetized iron bars protruded" (Inglis 1989:48).[10] Many of Mesmer's patients reported themselves cured. His services were in high demand. But he was denounced as a charlatan by his medical peers and finally by an international scientific committee convened by the French government (Gauld 1992).[11]

Generations later, Allen Kardec was himself an active member of the Mesmer Society of Paris, pursuing issues Mesmer had initiated, perhaps inadvertently incorporating aspects of Mesmer's philosophy into Spiritist thinking. The conviction that there were forces beyond the comprehension of conventional science reinforced belief in a spirit world and communication with it as part of treating human ills. Is it possible that producing some form of trance became part of Spiritist healing, providing the anesthesia essential for surgeries? If so, it must have been at a subliminal level. Kardec doesn't speak of or allude to it.

My thoughts drifted into word play: how could these patients become so "entranced" that they don't worry about being cut, so "mesmerized" that they feel no pain?

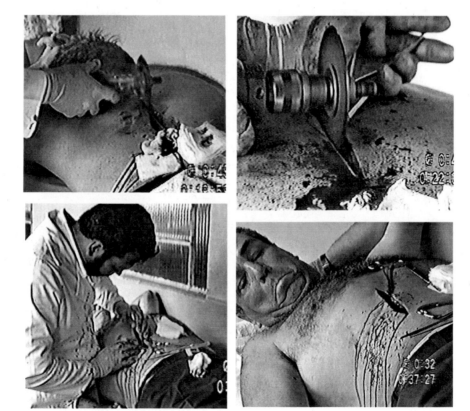

(Upper left) Antonio de Oliveira Rios/Dr. Stams cutting a patient's back with an electric saw. (Upper right) Close-up of Antonio de Oliveira Rios/ Dr. Stams cutting a patient's back with an electric saw. (Lower left) Antonio de Oliveira Rios/Dr. Stams making an incision in a patient's chest. (Lower right) Patient observing the incision made in his chest.

CHAPTER 4

MAURICIO MAGALHÃES IN CAMPO GRANDE

A decade later I was in Campo Grande, capital of the southwestern state of Mato Grosso do Sul, again seeing and hearing Dr. Fritz. This time he was incorporated in Mauricio Magalhães, a popular local healer.

My focus during this Brazilian sojourn was on the reactions of patients. I'd spoken with many of them over the years, interviewing some in their homes and others when they returned to a center to see a healer-medium for additional treatments. During one field trip, two U.S. physicians who were research colleagues of mine conducted some pre- and postsurgical examinations.

All this work confirmed that operations such as removing growths and scraping eyes had very high success rates without evident infections or postoperative complications. Surgeries performed not to deal directly with diseased or injured tissue but to give healing spirits access to the patient likewise produced few instances of negative side effects.

Almost all patients contacted believed they'd benefited, even those without unequivocal success. Sometimes this meant that death by cancer occurred several years later than predicted by conventional physicians, or that debilitating backaches were reduced enough to enable a return to work, or that a gravely depressed person could function again.

Professionals at seminars and conferences dealing with alternative and complementary medicine, and with what some are now calling subtle energies, saw my evidence as compelling, albeit incomplete. Yet those in mainstream medicine and its research establishment could shrug off the findings with the complaint that they were anecdotal. I realized that we needed "systematic studies." So in the summer of 1992, I undertook a survey of those receiving treatment from Mauricio Magalhães/Dr. Fritz.

I had met Mauricio the previous August when he was visiting Fortaleza to treat patients. Eleanor and I, plus two medical colleagues and several psychologists and anthropologists, had stopped there as part of an extended trip to observe healer-mediums. While he was invested with the persona of Dr. Fritz at the home of an affluent local industrialist suffering from an incurable disease, I asked if I could observe his work in Campo Grande, where he would be living the following summer. And could I interview his patients after their treatments? I anticipated rejection of what could have seemed an intrusion into his work, assessing its very efficacy. Mauricio, a somewhat chunky man with a round face, dark skinned and mostly bald, whose talk is restrained, steady, and deliberate even out of trance, displayed nothing like the youthful exuberance of José Carlos, the macho style of Antonio, or the jovial effusiveness of Edson.

He surprised me with his response: "I'm seeking to overcome the resistance I face in the scientific community to accepting what I have been reporting about Spiritist healers. Your help would be invaluable."

"That's very important! How else can we rescue them from their ignorance! You have a hard job," he added. "Those who fear the truth do not want to hear about it. You may interview my patients in Campo Grande."

The door was opened, although not as wide as I desired. I wanted to have physicians examine patients some months after their treatments.

"No, no. That is not workable, not possible. The arrangements would be too difficult. Besides, physicians must care for the ill, not devote a lot of time to those we've already cured."

Later, after Dr. Fritz had left him, Mauricio remained adamant. "You must do this yourself. I'm sure you'll find a way." Then he unintentionally suggested one.

"A year from now will be a very busy time for me. I'll be in the middle of my campaign for a seat on the city council."

That news didn't surprise me. Spiritists, like other religious leaders in Brazil, participated in politics on behalf of their interests, often trying to protect their right to pursue their unconventional practices. Edson Queiroz had won a seat in the legislature of the state of Pernambuco in 1989. Suddenly, I imagined an approach that could bring together my current concern with the outcomes of treatment by Spiritist healers with my long-standing interest in how underlying Brazilian cultural themes of patronage and clientage manifest themselves in electoral politics (Greenfield and Cavalcante 2006; Greenfield and Prust 1990; Greenfield 1979a, 1977b, 1972).

"Can a way be found for me to observe and participate in your campaign during the same time I observe your work as a healer and talk with some of those you treat?"

"Why not? Why not? You will find a way."

Finding the way required some invention and negotiation. Eleanor and I were working with a middle-aged woman named Maria de Lourdes Nardi, or Malú as she was known, who was a police officer in another state. She was one of a team of volunteers who'd established a Spiritist center in Campo Grande, a fast-growing frontier city of over 400,000. In addition to assisting Mauricio when he treated patients, she went out almost every afternoon to distant neighborhoods to visit those he'd attended and to urge them to vote for the medium. Another member of the team had organized on a computer the names and addresses of everyone registered for treatment by Dr. Fritz since Mauricio had returned from Fortaleza.

Accompanying Malú, we drove to the new neighborhoods of Campo Grande to interview ex-patients before she made her campaign pitch. These developments, unlike other parts of the city and the outlying areas of many of Brazil's urban centers, had sidewalks, electricity, water, and sewage lines. Their small, one-story houses were mostly brick with tile roofs, though some were wood and had thatched tops. Almost all the homes, usually built one room at a time, had refrigerators, TVs, and stereos with large, prominently displayed speakers.

Sheep, goats, and cows still grazed on the occasional empty lots. Most streets were unpaved, not yet on the map. Dust swirled up behind us. It coated everything, even the trees. Street signs were rare. Only a few of the one-story houses had numbers. It was harder to find the houses whose addresses we had than to get interviews—if and when the persons we sought were at home. By the end of this first day's foray, we'd completed only three interviews.

Malú asked the questions on our interview schedule. Eleanor audiotaped what was said while I videotaped the interviews and any conversations with us or with others who may have been present. Videos of the outside and inside of each dwelling reminded us of the family's social and economic standing. Once we felt secure about our schedule of questions and the interview process, Eleanor and I undertook some interviews on our own while Malú continued to do others. Sometimes it was necessary to return another day to find a former patient at home. Other volunteers in the healer's campaign group also did some interviews for us. After three arduous weeks we had completed thirty-two interviews.

I thought of surveys in the States, where academics are often able to field cadres of graduate assistants or turn the effort over to professional research organizations. Most of them do most of their interviews by telephone and mail. Their hundreds of respondents are selected randomly or in other ways to make them representative. Our thirty-two respondents will no doubt be designated, with implied disdain, a "convenience" sample, meaning that we took what we could get where we could get it. Better than "anecdotes"—but not much leverage for changing established convictions within the establishment.

So be it. My decades of experience with Spiritist healer-mediums and their patients convinced me that the responses of these individuals to the questions we'd asked would not change significantly within a large, scientifically selected sample, but I wished that an agency with the necessary resources would appear to test that conviction.

Because we went to outlying areas where Mauricio's volunteers were seeking potential voters, we didn't encounter his wealthier or higher status patients. Five of our respondents were unemployed. Eleven were housewives who didn't work outside the home. Three were self-employed. The others included factory workers, school custodians, domestic servants, retired persons, a high school teacher, an airline clerk, and a university student.

Some had a physician's diagnosis. The rest described their ailments as they had to Mauricio's assistants, designating the parts of their bodies where symptoms seemed to be experienced. Like those

I'd seen treated by José Carlos, Edson, and Antonio, some reported more than one problem or symptom. More than half spoke of pain—in the back, the throat, the stomach, the kidneys, the urinary tract, and in legs, knees, and joints. There were eye problems, hernias, bruises, swelling, sores, and bronchitis. By the last of our interviews, the total list included high cholesterol, prostate problems, gastritis, asthma, a stomach ulcer, impaired hearing, high blood pressure, rheumatism, anemia, bone cancer, enlarged veins, a growth on the head, and an infant with deformed feet.

Why did these thirty-two individuals with such a diverse array of problems, illnesses, and injuries seek help from Mauricio/Dr. Fritz? Twenty asserted that they knew someone who had been cured previously by Dr. Fritz. Thirteen had gone at the recommendation of a relative or friend. One was afraid of regular doctors, but nine others were moved by feelings of desperation at the failure of the licensed physicians from whom they'd sought help. Four were avowed Spiritists already convinced—as was the doctor from Rio who went to Recife—that healer-mediums provided the best treatments. Except for another four who said they had gone only out of curiosity, the rest were at least favorably disposed. All but two were convinced that spirits working through mediums could cure people and that Mauricio Magalhães was such a medium for Dr. Fritz.

Twenty-eight believed that they had been helped by their treatment; six did not. Twenty-one considered themselves cured. Of nineteen who said they had been treated for the same problem by a conventional doctor, all but one judged Dr. Fritz's treatment to be more successful. Twenty-nine said they would again seek help from Spiritist healers for future illness. Twenty-eight said they would recommend Mauricio/Dr. Fritz to others, and twelve said they would go only to him (see Greenfield 1997 for further details).

This is how the Spiritist movement continues to gather adherents, and how individual healer-mediums acquire their followings. Although many patients do not frequent Spiritist centers, attend sessions, or participate in rituals, they have learned and accepted something of Spiritist doctrine, which in this and other ways has infused into the larger culture.

At various times I watched Mauricio treat patients. He often employed invasive techniques. Yet he had his own way, his own style, and his own level of drama. When he used syringe needles, he moved very rapidly, going back and forth between several people as they reclined on three hospital gurneys or makeshift beds placed next to each other lengthwise. Three or four members of his team of assistants stood beside each.

He approached quickly, took 22-gauge syringe needles from their packaging, and thrust them into areas of complaint—often right through the patient's clothing. He neither asked questions nor listened to what patients said was wrong with them. It was assumed that Dr. Fritz already knew. The patient was left with up to five needles stuck into the back, abdomen, chest, throat, or wherever as Mauricio moved to the next person and the next before returning. He withdrew and rapidly reinserted the needles into other places before casually tossing them on the floor. Occasionally he told someone to turn over because he wanted to treat something about which the patient had not complained.

Even eyes did not escape the pervasive needles. Before treating a man's cornea, Mauricio inserted several needles at the edge of the eye, leaving them there while he treated other patients. Then he returned, removed the needles, and scraped the eye with a scalpel.

At times, considering a case to be especially serious, Mauricio/Dr. Fritz followed the use of needles with an incision adjacent to the spinal column about halfway down. Into this he inserted a hemostat or other blunt instrument, pushing it under the skin six to eight inches along the spine. The opening was intended to bring more energy from the spirit world to dematerialize growths or other objects whose presumed presence was thought to impede the normal functioning of the material body.

"Take hold of this," he often said to an onlooker, pointing to the half to two inches of the device left sticking out. "Pull it out."

Such a "volunteer" was usually someone whose interest and participation Mauricio wished to cultivate. A member of the team then covered the wound with ointment and a bandage.

"How did you feel when you were being treated?" each of the thirty-two respondents was asked.

Of the twenty-three who spoke about their emotions, fourteen admitted to being tense or afraid before seeing Mauricio. The other nine felt secure and calm. Twenty-nine made reference to pain—four to say that they felt some, four to assert that they felt only the prick of the needle, and eighteen to claim that they experienced no discomfort at all.

Late at night I sat in an otherwise dark room looking at the sheets of paper spotlighted under my desk lamp—tables of numbers displaying our respondents' answers. There would be excited, positive reactions among those I'd come to know back home and in other countries who also were exploring realms of human illness and wellness beyond the mainstreams of conventional biomedicine. And I could anticipate the dismissive challenges from critics: Proof? Where is the proof? Where are the pre- and post-treatment diagnoses by independent physicians? Where are the comparable samples using conventional treatments? How about replications?

Of course we could have done more with greater resources. But I'd finally realized that the problem of convincing those in the mainstream wasn't primarily one of funding or research techniques. It was much more profoundly a matter of how we viewed the world, what we believed about being human and about gaining knowledge of aspects of our humanity that lay beyond the reach of current scientific dogmas, as so much of my room lay beyond the circle of light on my desk.

CHAPTER 5

NOT ALL PATIENTS ARE CURED

KARDECISM'S APPROACH TO DEATH AND DYING

In 1981, while still in Fortaleza, I received an invitation from a man named Paulo Schutz, then director of the Graduate Program in Education of the Federal University of Rio Grande do Sul, to present a series of lectures. I soon learned that he had earned a PhD a few years previously at the University of Wisconsin at Madison. Having become disillusioned with the contribution that the exclusively quantitative techniques he had been taught could make to his understanding of the culture and society of the children he was training teachers to teach, he wanted me to speak to his faculty and students about the qualitative approaches employed in anthropology. I could not know at the time that this brief sojourn would bring me into ever more interesting aspects of Spiritist endeavors.

One of the members of the Faculty of Education who attended my lectures was a professor at the university named Cícero Marcos Teixeira, who also was a practicing Spiritist. Moreover, he had helped found, and at the time was the director of, an important Spiritist center; he also had written extensively on, and was extremely knowledgeable about, Spiritist thought. As a longtime friend of my host, he was present at the numerous social events Brazilians always combine with working visits. In the course of our conversations, I was able to discuss with him my growing interest in the belief system to which he had dedicated his life. Providing me with an extensive reading list, he invited me to visit his center and observe and videotape the healing activities. He also introduced me to other Spiritist intellectuals in the city whose work I later returned to study.

I had made plans with Professor Schutz to return to the state for a different research project that he and I were to undertake jointly. He was to spend a year with me in Milwaukee studying anthropology and its research methods. Afterward, we would conduct a collaborative study of German ethnicity and ethnic identity in Rio Grande do Sul, starting in the rural neighborhood where he had grown up and spoken German as his first language. A month before my new colleague was to arrive in the United States with his family, I received a letter from him. My vigorous, energetic friend had been stricken with cancer. Our plans had to be put on hold. In all our conversations, I had not spoken in any detail to Paulo of my work on healing. But when I learned of his illness, I immediately wrote to him about Spiritist healing and the healers' claims to be able to cure cancer. He replied that he already knew about Edson Queiroz and that Cícero had arranged for him to be treated when the healer made a visit to the nearby town of Novo Hamburgo. In February 1984, the licensed medical doctor from Recife who was a medium for Dr. Adolph Fritz and his team of disincarnate healers treated Paulo with the "advanced" facilities and techniques of the spirit world.

The treatment consisted of the insertion of needles by the medium into the area from which Paulo's colon had recently been medically removed. After going into trance, Edson/Dr. Fritz had taken a 22-gauge syringe needle from its original wrapping and jammed it rather forcefully into the region of the removed colon. He had not asked Paulo what was wrong with him and showed no interest when the patient tried to tell him. Dr. Fritz, according to the belief system and as we have seen, already knew, so there was no reason to ask or listen. In just a few seconds the needle was inserted and withdrawn, with the process repeated six times. Paulo later confided that all he felt was a series of pricks that did not hurt. Cícero explained that the treatment was intended to bring energy from the spirit world to dematerialize any cancer cells that had not been removed surgically and to help in the healing of the wounds. Paulo claimed that he felt stronger and better after the treatment. His oncologist encouraged him to continue with the Spiritist therapy even after he resumed chemotherapy.

Paulo had two more treatments by the spirits on Dr. Fritz's team in the winter of 1984. In what is called "treatment at a distance," they came to him at his home while he slept and provided the therapy they believed he needed. In reply to a letter sent by Cícero requesting the treatment, the volunteer staff at the center in Recife instructed Paulo to take a specified number of "passes," to attend an indoctrination session at a Spiritist center of his choice, and to eat or abstain from certain foods and activities for a specified period of days. On a designated night he was supposed to dress in white clothing and get into bed under white sheets before 7:00 p.m. A glass of water "fluidified" at a Spiritist center was to be placed next to him on his bed stand. He was to go to sleep, or lie perfectly still, but to awaken by 10:00 p.m., when he was to drink the water.

Paulo claimed to feel better after each treatment, although his condition in fact grew worse in the months to follow. Soon he was bedridden. His doctors could no longer offer hope. Instead they prescribed medications to ease the pain. His Spiritist friends continued to visit him at his home, where they pursued both further treatment and the "therapy" of further indoctrination into Spiritist beliefs.

Paulo was not a religious person. He was a classic example of what Robert Lowie was referring to when he said that to "the modern intellectual," which Paulo had become, "religion is probably the most unfamiliar subject in the world" (Lowie 1963:533). He thought of himself as a scientist. He believed science to be rational, while religion for him was based on superstition. He had been baptized as a child and had been taught the Brazilian variant of the German Catholic tradition of his forefathers. But as he advanced in school, he rejected the European-derived beliefs of his parents. He resented especially the Roman Catholic idea that illness was a punishment by God. By rejecting Catholicism, Paulo also cut himself off from whatever understanding and treatment options it offered that might enable him to cope with his imminent demise. And by substituting for it intellectual rationalism, he came to realize that he had opted for a system of beliefs that had little to offer on the subject he most needed to address. As one student of Spiritism has expressed it, "Science can answer many questions, but when faced with death and other ultimate problems of meaning, the scientific world view either responds with silence or suggests skepticism" (Hess 1993:ix). "Medical Science," adds Hall (1999), "has never truly come to grips with dying as a subject worthy of studying—the study of how it might be made more painless, more enriching." Coping with one's own death is instead left to the individual, to be thought about, if at all, in old age, supposedly after life is completed. But Paulo was not to live to an old age. His doctors, who acknowledged their "failure" in "losing" this vital and intelligent man, told him that he probably would not live to celebrate his fortieth birthday.

His colleagues did not know what to say to him. As is characteristic of educated Westerners, they were embarrassed when forced by circumstances to interact with him. Cícero Marcos Teixeira, on the contrary, sought out Paulo and offered not just his sympathy but also assistance. Shortly after the first (medical) surgery, at the request of Sueli, Paulo's wife, Cícero visited him in the hospital.

Over the years, Paulo had turned a proverbial deaf ear to Cícero's efforts to enlighten him about Spiritism. At Sueli's request, Cícero administered "hand passes" to bring healing energy from the other, or invisible, world to Paulo in the hospital. When the patient reluctantly admitted that he felt better after receiving them, Cícero returned daily for additional treatment. He also explained to Paulo how Spiritism interpreted and reacted to illnesses such as his. Paulo now understandably was more receptive and accepting than he had been previously. He listened attentively and read with interest the books Cícero left with him.

When Paulo was discharged from the hospital, Cícero came to his home, where he continued to administer passes not just to Paulo but also to Sueli and their children. He discussed Spiritist thinking with all of them. Soon, other Spiritist colleagues from the university formed a treatment group that in time came to meet weekly at the Schutz home. The group was organized and directed by a local medical doctor who was also a Spiritist. In their conversations, they outlined the fundamentals of the belief system. As Paulo's interest grew, they gave him more books to read.

In the spirit of a true researcher, Paulo volunteered to be part of my study of Spiritist healing. When I made arrangements to return to Recife for a second summer with Edson Queiroz/Dr. Fritz in

1984, Paulo said that he would also make the trip and asked me to register him for additional treatment. This task enabled me to go through the registration procedure and provided me with insights into what patients and their loved ones went through. In this case, I was registering a secular, rationalist university professor educated in the United States who—not unlike many readers of this book—adamantly opposed belief in any religion. I not only accompanied Paulo to his treatment but also taped interviews with him, during which he reflected on his feelings and emotional reactions. Moreover, as things turned out, I was able to accompany my friend's death and dying as part of and in the context of his family and loved ones through the lenses of Spiritist beliefs.

Spiritist healer-mediums, I had learned, did not cure all patients who came to them. For some people, an illness is believed to be part of the lesson they are to learn in their present incarnation.

After his second (medical) surgery, Paulo was placed on a regimen of chemotherapy. His Spiritist friends, meanwhile, urged him to visit a Spiritist center and seek independent treatment there.[12] Paulo broached the idea of treatment by the healer-medium to his oncologist. Since his chemotherapy had been suspended temporarily because the needed drugs were not available in Brazil, the doctor stated that he saw nothing wrong with his patient going to the *curendeiro*. Given the gravity of the situation, it probably could not hurt, he added. When the chemotherapy was completed, Paulo took homeopathic remedies prepared and dispensed at no cost at most Spiritist centers.

Spiritists believe in reincarnation. They postulate that spirits who move from one domain to another and back again in a series of limited stays drive the dual universe. The key to understanding this dynamic is Spiritism's view of evolution and progress in which the individual spirit is the basic unit. When God created the world, Kardec wrote, each spirit was set on a path of development that eventually will lead it to its moral and spiritual perfection.

The material world in this view is assumed to be something like an obstacle course, or perhaps a schoolhouse. It provides situations from which lessons may be learned. Spirits are assumed to return to the material world repeatedly, over the millennia, each time to learn a specific lesson, or set of lessons, that will move them along their developmental path. Eventually, when they master all needed lessons, they achieve a state of perfection and no longer must return to the material world.

Spiritism is a morally driven system of beliefs. Its standards derive from the Judeo-Christian tradition that Kardec intended to modify and revise. The exemplar of spiritual perfection for Spiritists is Jesus Christ, whom they see as neither the son of God nor the messiah but the most advanced spirit ever to have appeared on this planet. His life, his words, and his deeds set the standards for proper thought and conduct to which all touched by Spiritist thought are urged to aspire. Kardec interpreted and revised the Gospels to emphasize what he believed were Jesus's most important teachings (Kardec [1864] 1987).

The developmental progress of individual spirits may be hampered in two ways. First, in spite of intense deliberations and planning, by the time a spirit takes a physical body and grows to maturity, it often no longer remembers the lesson it has come back to learn. Second, spirits are assumed to have free will. Even when they do remember, they still may choose not to devote themselves to the mission they have incarnated to learn. Since they are not punished for not mastering what they have returned to undertake, at worst they must repeat the same lesson in the future. The role of indoctrination sessions is to impress on errant, misbehaving spirits the need to accept guidance that will redirect them to their intended tasks. Since coping with illness may be the lesson a spirit has returned to master, indoctrination is offered as part of most Spiritist healing sessions (see Greenfield 1993, 1992).

Paulo claimed that during the indoctrination sessions he attended, the lessons he was to learn in this incarnation became clear to him. While listening to lectures and reading, reflecting on, and discussing texts, he was able to see his particular situation in terms of the general principles of reincarnation, karma, and spiritual development. He understood that his illness was part of the lesson he had come back to learn. With the help of messages transmitted through mediums from guides on the other plane, he realized that it would be counterproductive for him to be cured. He was made aware that he had completed most other aspects of his mission. While he might delay his "departure" a bit longer for the sake of his family, colleagues, and friends, it really was time for him to move on along on his inevitable path.

This reasonable and proper choice (according to Spiritist teaching) was made more inviting to Paulo by accounts he read of life on the other plane. Spiritist publications, such as the classic *Nosso Lar* (Xavier 1944), often include reports given to mediums by spirits wishing to inform the living of what life is like in the other world. Paulo learned that on the spirit plane he would be able to live the life of learning and reflection he so loved. There was music and art and time for sociability with friends and loved ones. He could study and conduct research. Certainly, he would miss his parents, wife, children, and friends, but he would be able to remain in communication with them for the remainder of each of their lives in the material world, and in time they would join him. Spirits, he learned, tend to travel together in groups in their many incarnations. Members of the same family and others with strong attachments are said to return to the material plane together. While their relationships may differ each time, with a father in one lifetime being the son in another (reversing the parent–child relationship), a spouse becoming a student or a friend of the same sex, a friend an enemy, or a lover an adversary, they will be in the same place at the same time and be able to meet and interact. For Paulo, this meant that he would see us all either on the spirit plane or in this world at some time in the future.

Paulo Schutz departed the material world on a Saturday afternoon in 1985. Present at his home at the time were his wife, children, parents, relatives, and Spiritist friends who were still meeting with him, now more to teach and help him with the transition than to treat him. One of them later told me that the group had arrived at about 11:00 a.m. When they entered Paulo's bedroom, his spirit already had separated from his physical body. Although he was still talking lucidly, when the mediums went into trance, the voices of the spirits they received came from a direction other than the one where Paulo's material body lay. When they left the room, they agreed to wait near a telephone for a call informing them that the end was at hand. The call came at about four in the afternoon.

Paulo believed that his wife would be strong, independent, and able to provide the emotional support and guidance that their children would need to grow up and learn about their places in the world, their missions, and how best to accomplish them. Before their intensive study of Spiritism during his illness, Paulo did not know whether Sueli had that ability. By the time he was ready to disincarnate, he was convinced that she did.

Paulo no longer feared the end of his life on earth and knew it to be a part of a "cosmic reality" that now made sense to him. This understanding—the teachings about reincarnation, the dual universe, the role of spirits, their need for development, and, perhaps most important, the belief that he would travel over the millennia accompanied by his loved ones—provided him with a peace and sense of tranquility and security, something he had not had during the months of struggle after being diagnosed with a terminal illness.

This may explain the following incident that took place several years after his death. In 1988 I was back in Porto Alegre on another Fulbright award, teaching this time in the Department of Anthropology at the Federal University of Rio Grande do Sul. I had taken some of my students to observe the weekly healing activities by Dr. José Lacerda—whom we will meet shortly—and his Casa do Jardim healing group. Paulo's wife, Sueli, also joined me that morning. She had taken the "learning-disabled" son of the man with whom she was now living to see if Dr. Lacerda might be able to help him.

In the late morning, my wife came to take me from a room in which I was observing Dr. Lacerda to another room, where a medium was already in trance. When I arrived, the spirit she had incorporated was addressing Sueli, the boy, and his father in what sounded to all of us like Paulo's voice. (As soon as my wife had heard the voice, she had come to find me. My students, I should note, were not quite sure what to make of it all.) After a lengthy message to Sueli in which, among other things, he expressed his approval of her decision to live with the boy's father, he said that he had a message for Sid. Of my very large number of Brazilian friends, including those who have spent time in the United States, Paulo was one of the very few to call me Sid, as opposed to Sidney, or "*Doutor*, Professor," or "*Senhor*" Sidney (usually pronounced *Sídg ni*) or Sid (pronounced *Sídg*).

The message to me was simple. Paulo just wanted me to know that there would be plenty of opportunity for us to conduct collaborative research in the spirit world. He would be waiting for me no matter when I arrived. There was no need for me to rush.

In the more than two and one-half decades since Paulo's death, Sueli and the children have managed. She has become a strong and vibrant person who has maintained her home and family, often in the face of considerable adversity. Certainly she and the children have missed Paulo and feel that their lives would have been richer and more complete were he still here. But without him, they have not fallen into despair. They have come to see his death as related to what they are here on earth to accomplish. Spiritism, it appears, has helped the whole family cope with death and living.

CHAPTER 6

THE DISOBSESSION

ANOTHER FORM OF SPIRITIST THERAPY

At the turn of the twentieth century, Dr. Adolfo Bezerra de Menezes Cavalcanti, a medical doctor, proposed a novel theory to explain mental illness. Originally from Fortaleza, he had moved to the then national capital Rio de Janeiro to study. After earning his degree, he remained there to practice and later entered politics. Bezerra, who had treated mental patients in Rio jails, read Kardec's writings soon after they were translated into Portuguese and became a convert to his thinking (see Acquarone 1982; Soares 1962). As a leading local advocate of the new doctrine, he adopted Kardec's belief that mental illness, in the absence of lesions on the brain, was caused by spirits. While some spirits intended to harm their victims, most were simple, decent beings who, on disincarnating, "were confused." With their material bodies no longer available and functional for them—often already placed in the ground—they sought a second body, attempting to continue living in or through it even though it was already occupied by another incarnate being. Kardec had used the term *obsession* to refer to the behavioral effects of situations in which two spirits temporarily competed for the use of the same body. Conventional medicine, meanwhile, assuming consistency in the behavior of the individual over time, categorized the situation as mental illness. To treat it, Bezerra proposed that the offending spirit be "rehabilitated," by which he meant explaining to it that it must go off to the spirit world and prepare for its next incarnation, enabling the "owner" of the body temporarily inhabited by two spirits to return to the status quo ante, or what is medically defined as normalcy. Bezerra called the procedure for removing the obsessing spirit a disobsession (see also Franco 1979).

Bezerra and others who applied this therapeutic technique found that offending spirits, once reminded (or advised) of the inappropriateness of their actions and set back on the road to development, eventually would stop what they were doing. Most of those they were obsessing would cease experiencing symptoms of (mental) illness.

Additional forms of treatment were added to the Spiritist healing repertory when other Brazilian Spiritist intellectuals, using Kardec's technique of asking enlightened spirits in the other world (through mediums if they did not have the ability themselves), obtained further information about the workings of the universe. Spirits of deceased doctors, such as Fritz and Stams, and of other healers presently in the other plane, such as St. Ignatius, were asked—or in some cases volunteered—to cooperate in the treatment of the living. Mediums would relay the symptoms of patients to the spirit doctors, who would make diagnoses and recommend treatments, at times prescribing medications, both allopathic and homeopathic, and other forms of therapy.

While some Spiritist healers treated only patients with mental problems, others, wishing to help those with physical illnesses, elaborated healing by the spirits in two other directions. One group developed techniques by which the several bodies they assumed a human being to be composed of—such as the material or the spiritual—could be separated, so that at least one would be "transported" to the spirit plane. There, previously contacted spirit doctors attend to them. Diagnosis and treatment usually require the reconstruction of aspects of one or more of the patient's previous lives to determine the cause of the present symptoms. Treatment consists of convincing a spirit who has been harmed or injured by the spirit of the patient in a previous lifetime and is now seeking revenge, which is the immediate cause of the patient's symptoms, to stop what it is doing (see Greenfield 1993, 1992).

Another group approached spirits of deceased doctors and healers and invited them to return temporarily to the material plane to treat incarnate patients. For reasons related to their individual spiritual development, some accepted the offer. These disincarnate spirits, including Drs. Fritz and Stams and St. Ignatius, are assumed to "take over" (in a form of spirit possession) the body of the medium through whom they work to offer a range of medical and surgical options. In both cases, illness considered to be physical by conventional medicine may be treated with Spiritist techniques.

Most believers in Spiritism accept the idea that germs, viruses, and microbes cause disease. They go to doctors, take prescribed medications, and submit to surgeries and other recommended procedures. In addition, they believe in analogous things in the spirit world that make spirits sick. If spirit doctors do not treat these "illnesses" with spirit surgeries or spirit medications before the next spirit incarnates, the illnesses will be carried along and appear materially in the new body. Spiritists believe in a symbiotic relationship between the spirit and the physical body it will use each time it returns to the material world. Uncured illnesses from previous lifetimes (in either world) are believed to cause some of the illnesses experienced by incarnate beings. Medical treatment alone cannot cure them. Once they are diagnosed, treatment by a healer-medium with access to the therapies of the spirit world is necessary. Spiritist therapy, consequently, must complement medical treatment, if not replace it altogether.

Almost three-quarters of a century after Bezerra first formalized the disobsession, I visited a Spiritist center in Rio de Janeiro noted for helping those in need of this treatment. It was 2:00 p.m. on a hot summer afternoon. The heavy iron gate on a street in an upscale neighborhood had just been locked. Several hundred people inside the gate were making their way up a steep hill to a large building at the top. Within minutes they were seated on benches in a room resembling a lecture hall. At the front was a table, around which eight people dressed in white were seated. A man standing at a microphone offered a testimonial. He explained how the spirits had helped him recover from a debilitating illness. (Patients who wait for treatments by José Carlos, Edson, Antonio, and Mauricio hear similar testimonials.) While his story was meaningful, even inspiring, his voice, and that of other speakers to follow, was soft and tedious. It showed no change of pitch or emotion.

To the right of the table was a room, where eighteen to twenty individuals stood, each facing an empty chair. Off to the side was yet another, even smaller space, with several healers standing behind a curtain. In contrast with the stark whiteness of the previous rooms, this one had an altar covered with brightly colored statues and other items.

The more than three hundred individuals seated quietly in the lecture hall were multiracial, of both sexes and all ages, but the majority were white females. Less than a third were men, a still smaller percentage black. The approximately seventy-five children sat motionless, hardly uttering a sound during the lengthy session.[13] The male at the microphone continued his presentation for some minutes, followed by a well-dressed woman, who affirmed with her own tale the power of the spirits and how they had cured her. By then, after listening to such stories during visits to other centers, I understood that they were standard procedure at all forms of Spiritist healing. For exactly one hour, the audience listened attentively as a succession of believers delivered soliloquies in similar soft, dry, monotonous styles about their own healings by spirits. The final speaker formally opened the session by invoking God, Christ, and the saints, asking for their help in the work to be undertaken. The spirits of the dead were entreated to cooperate. After reading several prayers, taken mostly from the Christian Gospels, the man invited Ogun and other African deities to assist in the venture. He led the audience in special songs, each intended to summon the participation of a specific African-derived supernatural.[14] Meanwhile, the people seated around the table, who appeared to be paying no attention to what those at the microphone were saying or doing, were busily engrossed in automatic writing—reminiscent of how José Carlos, Edson, Antonio, and Mauricio wrote prescriptions when in trance—their eyes gazing blankly into the distance.

At precisely 3:00 p.m., the person at the microphone stopped talking. Groups of about twenty individuals at a time were led out of the lecture hall and seated in the chairs in the smaller room, facing healers dressed in white. With soft music playing in the background, others gave "healing passes"—intended to bring energy from the other, or spirit, world—to the newcomers. By 3:30 everyone was back in the lecture hall, where they picked up personal items that had been left unattended on the benches.

From 3:30 to 4:00 p.m., the cleansing continued. The hall and those in it were first bathed in smoke from a censer and then covered with rose petals. Precisely at 4:00 p.m., the day's major activity began. Ushers came to selected individuals and conducted them, one at a time, to still another large room. There, each person joined one of five groups of white-clad individuals who stood waiting for them. Those escorted were the patients; they had registered for treatment when they first arrived at the center earlier in the day. Those who remained behind in the main hall were their parents, children, relatives, and friends.

Every newcomer wanted to relate the symptoms for which relief was sought, but the healers, seemingly disinterested, quickly and quietly entered into trance. Almost immediately, one medium began to scream in pain and roll on the floor while a colleague bent over him as if he were performing surgery in the pelvic area. But this time there was no cutting. Like the placebo surgeries in the United States, it was all simulated. It soon became apparent that the exaggerated pantomime was of an abortion, but the patient being treated was a male.

As the medium in trance bent over his colleague in pain on the floor, a third person joined them. Fernando was a learned teacher of Kardec's philosophy and a leader at the center who circulated from group to group. When he arrived, he took over the direction of the therapeutic ritual. The others deferred to his authority. First he explained to the bewildered patient that in a previous lifetime he had been a woman who had aborted a life she had conceived illicitly. Kardecists believe that abortion is the taking of a life and oppose it as immoral. The cause of the symptoms the patient was experiencing—excruciating abdominal pains for which the doctors could find neither cause nor cure—was the spirit of the fetus who, as the result of the abortion, had been denied an opportunity to reincarnate and had chosen to devote itself to gaining revenge. Although the spirit that had prevented the incarnation by having the abortion was now in a male body, the aggrieved spirit was making it suffer the pains of the abortion for what it had done in a previous lifetime. Once the patient understood this, the leader explained, his treatment could begin.

As the patient stood there with his eyes slightly glazed over and a perplexed look on his face, Fernando, although he was not in trance, invoked and greeted the spirit of the aborted fetus, who appeared through another member of the group. "Hello," said Fernando, in a warm and friendly tone.

"Where am I?" exclaimed an unfamiliar voice coming from this other medium, who had distanced himself physically from the rest of the group. "Why am I here? I don't like it here. It is much too bright. What do you want with me?"

"Relax, take it easy," responded Fernando calmly. "I only wish to talk with you."

"I don't want to talk with you," responded the voice angrily. "I don't like it here. I wish to leave."

Fernando persisted, calmly reassuring the spirit and continuing to ask it questions. Although the other remained reluctant, repeating its desire to depart, it soon was caught up in conversation. The answers to the questions Fernando asked, some of which he provided himself when the spirit refused to respond, resulted in a dialogue that set out in summary form the basic beliefs and premises of Brazilian Kardecist-Spiritism.

First the spirit was reminded of the two orders of the cosmos. Gradually it was forced by the persuasiveness of Fernando's reasoning to agree that the advancement and moral progress of the individual (spirit) took precedence over all other matters. It admitted that it was presently disincarnate, meaning it was in the invisible world and not in a material body. In such a form, it acknowledged, it should not be interacting with the incarnate, especially by inflicting pain on them. It agreed that instead of taking vengeance on someone in the material world, which according to Kardec ([1864] 1987) also is immoral, it should concentrate on its own development by preparing to reincarnate.

The exchange between Fernando and the disincarnate being was at times quite heated. The latter tried to challenge and refute the assertions of faith made by his interlocutor, who would counter with a combination of eloquence and clear thinking. Occasionally, the protagonists' voices were raised as if in anger. Other times, one or the other responded in a whisper. In the end, the wrongdoing spirit was won over by the uncontestable "truth and logic" of Fernando's argument. The treatment for the patient's symptoms was the rehabilitation of a disincarnate spirit that had behaved inappropriately by seeking revenge. When finally convinced that what it was doing was morally wrong, and harmful to both the patient and itself, the reluctant spirit agreed to stop tormenting its nemesis, return to the spirit world, and prepare to reincarnate. The patient, dazed and confused by the events he had witnessed, was left only to anticipate that his pains would now disappear.

His treatment, which was the rehabilitation of a spirit that had been aggrieved by the patient in a previous lifetime and had inappropriately sought revenge, was between Fernando and the spirit. The patient seemingly took no part in the therapeutic ritual that was intended to benefit him. Unlike patients on whom surgeries are performed, who are the focus of the attention of loved ones and observers when operated on, here the patient stood by watching and listening to what was being done on his behalf with glazed eyes and a look of disbelief on his face. Only after the spirit that was the cause of his suffering had agreed to stop inflicting the pain and departed, and the mediums had come out of trance, was he addressed directly. Fernando told him that he now would be well and instructed him to read and reflect on the writings of Allan Kardec and other Spiritist authors, and as often as possible to attend sessions at a Spiritist (or Umbanda) center, where he should regularly obtain therapeutic passes.

I wondered as he departed how the young man had internalized what had happened, especially what Fernando had said by way of explanation. Did it make sense to him? Would he undergo any transformative experience? More importantly, would his pains now abate? I reflected on the fast and dramatic qualities of the surgeries as opposed to the slow theatrics of the disobsession ritual. I tried to connect them, to process the effects of each on the patients, and to process the implications for my understanding of Spiritist therapeutics. Since this center did not take names and addresses of those treated, I was unable to locate the patient to interview him after his treatment was completed.

Sometime later, in Porto Alegre, I attended other disobsession sessions directed by Dr. José Lacerda de Azevedo, a physician. The group that he led, Casa do Jardim, had begun in a small house (*casa*) in the (*do*) garden (*jardim*) of the local Spiritist hospital, hence the name. (In addition to their own healing as charity, Spiritists frequently support hospitals in which conventional treatments are provided.)

At 7:00 a.m. on a cold, wet Saturday morning, more than one hundred people lined up outside yet another Spiritist center where the group now practiced. Most of those waiting were from the greater Porto Alegre metropolitan area, but some had traveled from as far away as Brasília, the northeast, and Amazonas. A few had come from neighboring Uruguay and Argentina. The patients were suffering from illnesses as varied as cancer, depression, and drug addiction. The vast majority, unlike those treated in Recife, Fortaleza, Palmelo, Campo Grande, and Rio de Janeiro, appeared to be descendants of Europeans and of the middle and lower-middle socioeconomic classes. The poor (mostly black), so numerous in Porto Alegre and throughout the country, were conspicuously absent. Accompanied by friends and relatives, the patients—as young as ten and as old as eighty-five—had come to be treated by Dr. Lacerda and his associates of the Casa do Jardim.

At exactly 8:00 a.m., when the doors to the building were opened, those outside, whose numbers by then had more than doubled, were led into an auditorium. At the front, in an almost stereotypical dry and unemotional tone, a man recounted his story of how the spirits had healed him—a story that might be thought of as the preamble to all Spiritist treatment rituals. He was followed by a series of others, who presented their testimonials until Dr. Lacerda took the microphone. He offered a short prayer, in which he asked the cooperation of God, Christ, and the spirits in the work that was about to be undertaken. With the efficiency and resolve that characterized most Spiritist healing groups, members broke up into teams of four to seven persons, with each going to a different, smaller room. The same individuals tended to work together week after week. Everyone else waited in the assembly hall, listening to another series of believers somberly chronicling their cures by the spirits. As each patient's registration number was called, an escort took him or her to an assigned room.

I followed Dr. Lacerda that morning to what looked like a classroom. He went to a table with a blackboard at the front. The six members of his team took places along the sidewall. Several visitors learning the procedure sat near the leader. I was at the opposite sidewall with my notebook, video equipment, and tape recorder. The doctor greeted everyone individually as they entered and offered some general words of advice to the visitors. Then the first patient, a young woman, accompanied by her sister, entered. Both were invited to sit at the back of the room.

Lacerda asked if they were Spiritists. He followed their negative reply by inquiring if they had knowledge of the writings of Allan Kardec, Chico Xavier, or other Spiritist authors popular in Brazil. The patient responded that she had heard of the authors but had not read any specific books. Lacerda smilingly replied that perhaps she should begin to read and study. He invited her to present her problem to the group.

After a few minutes, group member Dr. Ivan Hervé, an elderly internist, politely interrupted to ask a question. The reply led to a brief exchange. It culminated in Dr. Hervé saying that it appeared that the patient had a thyroid problem that could easily be brought under control by conventional medicine. The type of treatment provided by this group was not needed, he said. On behalf of the group, he was eliminating the more common medical problems. He told the woman that she should go to a conventional physician if she had one, or else she could see him at his clinic.

Lacerda concurred with his colleague. He explained to the patient and the visitors that unlike other places where Spiritist healing was conducted, these sessions were devoted to assisting people with problems for which the medical establishment had no solutions. He suggested that she take Dr. Hervé's advice while reminding her to read classic Spiritist texts and learn some basic doctrine. After politely thanking everyone, the two women left the room.

The second patient was a well-dressed woman in her late thirties, accompanied by a distinguished-looking man wearing an expensive leather coat who introduced himself as her husband. When they responded "no" to the routine question about being Spiritists and familiarity with Spiritist literature, Lacerda repeated the recommendation he had made to the previous patient.

The woman then launched into her story. For the past several months, Anna recounted, she had been experiencing debilitating headaches and was suffering from excruciating pains in her back and legs. Although she had seen several doctors, the medications prescribed had not helped and the pain had increased.

Suddenly, Lacerda interrupted her, not to ask a question but to shout the word *plataforma* (platform). He began to count backward, rather loudly, while waving a metal rod over his head. He brought the rod down and then up, punctuating each number. After a few counts, a dark-haired woman seated at the side of the room began to speak in a voice very different from the one she had used previously. She had gone into trance and was describing a series of events in a past life of the patient. Anna, meanwhile, was so deep in conversation with Dr. Hervé that she appeared disinterested in what was happening around her.

According to Spiritist belief, immediately after conception, a reincarnating spirit attaches itself to the newly formed fetus by means of what is called its perispirit. This semimaterial, bioplasmic substance is believed to be a permanent part of every spirit and remains its link with the material body throughout each incarnation.

The chakras of the perispirit must be brought into line exactly with the plexus of the somatic body, uniting the otherwise separate domains of the universe (Greenfield 1987a). When this happens, a symbiotic relationship is established between the spirit and its material body.

Spiritism teaches that each living person is composed minimally of three distinct bodies: one spiritual, a second perispiritual, and the third material. Lacerda writes of seven, two material and five spiritual (Lacerda de Azevedo 1988:29–45). It is the last of the five spirit bodies, the astral, that is of special interest to us, since Lacerda and the Casa do Jardim healers believe it can be transported to the spirit world, separate from the rest of a patient's bodies, on the (invisible) platform he had previously invoked. There, Lacerda claims to have entered into a "contractual agreement" with a Dr. Lourenço, the director of the hospital Amor e Caridade (Love and Charity).

This was the destination to which Anna's astral body had been sent. It was also where the astral body of the medium who had reported an incident in the patient's past life had gone. As this incident was being shown on a large screen in the hospital in the spirit world, the medium reported it simultaneously to those of us at the Casa do Jardim.

After hearing her first few words, Lacerda turned to the visitors and exclaimed: "*Magia negra*" (black magic). A second medium, also at the hospital in the spirit world, took over. He described a scene in which the spirit that now occupied Anna's body inflicted a great injustice on a spirit that was presently incarnate as Marta, her sister-in-law. The two women had been enemies since both joined their husbands' family. The medium reported Marta swearing that she would get revenge.

Suddenly, a third medium opened his eyes and in a weak, crackling voice, very different from his usual baritone, uttered, "Where am I? How did I get here?"

Taking control of the situation, Lacerda, like Fernando, turned to the voice to reassure it. "*Calma* [relax]," he said, "we only wish to talk to you."

"I don't want to talk to you," replied the voice. "Let me go. I don't want to be here. I don't like it here! It is so bright! My eyes hurt! I want to go! Leave me alone!"

Lacerda persisted. "Would you not prefer to come out of the dark and leave the grime and filth? Don't you want to give up those ugly claws and the dirty fur?"

"No," snapped the voice, repeating that it did not want to be there or continue the conversation. Ignoring this, Lacerda asked further questions, gradually drawing the reluctant spirit into a dialogue. Like Fernando in the previous example, he cajoled and manipulated the spirit into acknowledging the Kardecist view of the world and its moral perspective. But there was something different: Lacerda made repeated references to low, heavy, base vibrations, claws, and fur and called the spirit variously a ghoul and a monster.

At one point, Lacerda called it an *exu*. Exus are part of the supernatural pantheon of Umbanda, said by some to have been brought from Africa by the slaves. Originally they were messengers to the *orixás*, the African deities. In Brazil, the African tradition was syncretized, first with Christianity to form Candomblé, Xangô, and Batuque (see chapter 9), and then with Spiritism to become Umbanda (see chapter 10). The exus in Umbanda have become a separate category of supernatural beings. They incorporate in mediums and, along with *pretos velhoss* (old former slaves), *caboclos* (Indians), and *crianças* (children), do the charity of helping people that Umbanda has taken from Kardecism to be its primary mission (Brown [1986]

1994; Greenfield and Prust 1990; Giobellina and Martinez 1989; Greenfield and Gray 1988; Pressel 1974).[15]

Kardecist mediums do not usually receive African-derived spiritual beings. They consider the religions of African provenience to be less enlightened than their own, and their deities to be lower forms. Along the continuum that was proposed to organize the variety of popular Brazilian religions (Bastide 1978), Kardecism, or *mesa branca* (white table) as it sometimes is called, has been placed at the highest end, and Candomblé, Xangô, Batuque, and the other heavily African-influenced religions at the lowest. Umbanda is somewhere between the extremes, said to be more advanced than those of strict African derivation but less so than Spiritism.

Unlike most Kardecists, Lacerda and the Casa do Jardim group acknowledge African-derived spirits that they believe are able to inflict illness and injury. By "encompassing" the discourse of Umbanda (see Hess n.d.), they are able to treat the illnesses caused by these "denser, less enlightened beings." Lacerda had encouraged and then arranged for several mediums in his group to join Umbanda centers, where they learned to incorporate its spirits. Thus in the session being described, a medium was able to receive the exus that seemed to be the cause of Anna's suffering.

When the spirit, after being convinced of Kardecism's basic truths, still refused to stop tormenting Anna, Lacerda authoritatively demanded that it tell him the name of its "boss." First denying that it took orders from anyone, the spirit eventually acquiesced.

A fourth medium, who had been sitting quietly all this time, now burst forth in a tirade and protested being in such a brightly lit place. A repeat of the earlier performance followed, with Lacerda, using the ritualized question-and-answer format, forcing the "boss" to acknowledge the moral truths of Spiritism and to admit the wrong he had done. The spirit confessed that he was not working alone but had a gang of underlings to whom he gave orders. Some time ago, he said, the spirit that was now incarnate as Marta had approached him and asked him to help her obtain revenge. One of his henchmen, acting on his instructions, had placed a tiny electronic device in Anna's head, causing the headaches and pains in her back and legs. The apparatus that only he was able to remove was connected to controls in his possession.

"This is the black magic I mentioned," Lacerda told the visitors. He explained that malevolent spirits are frequently organized in gangs, the leaders of which were once incarnate in ancient Egypt, the home of the black arts. Many, like the ones that appeared that day, had not reincarnated since. Instead of seeking new lives that would give them the opportunity to advance morally, they hid in the lowest, darkest, densest regions of the spirit world—known as the Umbral—and sold their services to other unenlightened spirits like the one now in the body of Marta.

After meekly acknowledging the errors of its ways, the boss spirit agreed to remove the apparatus, go to the "hospital" Amor e Caridade, and seek treatment and guidance that would enable him to reincarnate and pursue his spiritual development.

Turning away from the departing spirit, Lacerda muttered, *"Abrir a frequencia"* (open the frequency) and began to count backward, again accentuating each number with a wave of the metal rod. The first medium—who had accompanied Anna to the spirit plane and had been silent during the exchange with the two monster spirits—began to speak, this time in a voice different from either of those she had used before. She was joined by the only medium who had not yet spoken. They recounted the episode—now appearing to them on the screen in Dr. Laurenço's hospital—in which the spirit of Anna committed the original injustice against Marta. As the story unfolded, Lacerda made explicit to the patient the offense she had committed. He explained to the other spirit that although she had suffered an injustice, she should not have sought revenge. By means of the ritualized dialogue, he brought both spirits to concur that they each had been wrong, thus enabling him to propose that they now forget the past and devote themselves to their respective spiritual developments.

The spirit of Marta acknowledged her treachery and apologized. She ordered the black magician to have the apparatus removed. Finally, she implored the spirit of Anna to pardon her. In a scene filled with emotion, both spirits—more precisely the mediums incorporating them—begged the other for forgiveness. A lengthy embrace and a flood of tears marked the reconciliation. As the spirits departed the mediums, Lacerda raised his metal rod once more and again counted backward. Although the treatment was complete,

Anna's astral body had not yet been brought back from the hospital in the spirit world and rejoined with her other bodies. The medium standing next to her began applying hand passes to bring energy from the spirit world to facilitate the recoupling process. He also confirmed that all the devices had been removed. When he indicated that he was finished, Lacerda authoritatively pronounced that the patient would now be well. [16]

The incarnate Anna, meanwhile, was still engrossed in conversation with Dr. Hervé, the one member of the healing team—besides Dr. Lacerda—who had not gone into trance. She seemed to have been fully aware of the dramatic events played out before her but had not reacted and appeared somewhat dissociated. It was as if she was having difficulty comprehending what she had seen and heard and relating it to herself and her suffering.

Sensing her confusion, Lacerda assured Anna that she soon would have relief from the headaches and other pains. Without further explanation, he again instructed her to read the writings of Spiritist authors and to attend sessions at a Spiritist or Umbanda center on a regular basis. Finally, he informed her that she had mediumistic abilities and that she should develop them by taking training that would enable her to become a part of the Spiritist enterprise of doing healing and other charitable works. As Anna left the room on the arm of her husband—who also appeared confused and bewildered by what he had observed and heard—she expressed her deep gratitude to Dr. Lacerda and the members of the group.

Unable to find out what had happened from the perspective of the patient, who returned to Buenos Aires after the session, I later discussed the events with Dr. Hervé in a series of lengthy interviews. He elaborated that he and the others undertook this unconventional form of treatment only to help patients suffering from illnesses for which conventional medicine was not (yet) able to provide adequate treatment. I asked him how he and his colleagues could be sure that the symptoms of patients such as Anna would actually disappear, that they would be cured. At first he seemed uncertain as to how to answer me. After a few minutes, he replied that it really was no different from what happened when a patient left his or another doctor's office after being treated for a commonly known illness. Doctors assume their patients will recover because of the large number of comparable instances in which the treatment had been applied successfully in similar cases in the past. There is a long history, with large volumes of carefully documented evidence, that certain treatments help with specific illnesses, he responded. There are trials and tests employing extensive statistical analysis. We spoke about the need to acknowledge what was being done as treatment by this group and to evaluate whether it was efficacious. I suggested that to convince his medical colleagues of the value of the Spiritist treatments it would be necessary to document treatments, descriptions of symptoms being responded to, and follow-ups with patients to confirm their recovery. That would take time away from treatment, he protested. "We are all so busy, and there are so many people who need our help!" But as a trained scientist who had done a rotation in the United States, I argued, you know that it is necessary if you wish to convince scientific audiences of the value of what you are doing.

Many years later, when I returned to Porto Alegre on another matter, Dr. Hervé approached me at the home of a mutual friend to thank me. He also invited me to visit the new Spiritist center he had founded—after Dr. Lacerda's death—to show me the reams of case materials he had accumulated to document treatments conducted. He presented me with copies of several books in which he had published a sample of the results of this undertaking (Hervé 2006, 2004, 1999, 1996; Hervé et al. 2003). The published case materials contained descriptions of the symptoms of each patient, the treatment provided, and a follow-up presenting the outcome. Some of the reported cases involved what are called psychosomatic illnesses, while others were strictly somatic. The results were consistent with my own (Greenfield 1997) and Lynch's (1996) findings that patients reported high levels of successful treatment by healer-mediums who performed surgical in addition to the other interventions (see also Carvalho 1996, 1995). What was added by the work of Drs. Lacerda and Hervé, the Casa do Jardim, Hervé's Casa de João Pedro, the group in Rio de Janeiro, and the many others throughout the country is that interventions other than prescribing medications and performing surgery are employed with considerable success by Spiritist healers to help the suffering.[17]

Healers and patients in all of forms of Spiritist therapy do not necessarily share a cosmology, values, contexts, and systems of semiosis.

Most of those to seek help are not Spiritists, nor do they know and accept Spiritist beliefs before arriving at the facility where treatment is provided. Most patients learn the specifics of the belief system's view of the world for the first time as they wait for treatment. Specific teaching, especially during disobsession rituals, is directed at spirits not present in incarnate form. The patient is seemingly an outsider in this drama—in contrast with the surgeries, where the patient is part of the drama. Although being acted on, the patient stands by watching as others provide relevant information, heretofore unknown, about his or her past life experiences that serves as the bases for the indoctrination that convinces the offending spirit to depart. The uninvolved patient departs the disobsession appearing confused and bewildered. This situation makes it difficult to apply standard forms of anthropological analysis of ritual healing, which focus on the symbols knowingly shared by patient and healer, to understanding this Brazilian therapeutic endeavor. If healing is assumed to be the result of a transformation that a sick person undergoes during the course of the performance of a healing ritual, how do we explain how those treated in a disobsession move from a sick to a healthy state? I have hypothesized that the patients, as the magicians and my anesthesiologist friend pointed out after seeing the videos of the surgeries, are, like the mediums, in a trance or altered state of consciousness similar to hypnosis. But if it is true, how are they induced into the state? More importantly, how can this idea help explain the patients' not experiencing pain, absence of infections, and, most importantly, recovery?

CHAPTER 7

HEALING AND THE COMPETITION FOR RELIGIOUS CONVERTS

Dr. Edson Queiroz, his face always tight when he was host to the persona of Dr. Fritz, now displayed real anger. He literally shouted at me, "My patients are neither hypnotized nor mesmerized! The medium is in trance—to receive the spirits. The patients are not!"

I was back in Recife at Edson's Spiritist center. I had just asked Dr. Fritz, when he had stopped to answer questions after finishing with the last of the patients before leaving Edson's body (as was his custom), if the patients were in trance. During my return home to the United States, I had worked with members of the American Society for Clinical Hypnosis, sitting in on their introductory course for qualified professionals, mainly health care providers. I now knew why some magicians who saw my videotapes believed the patients undergoing surgeries were in a trancelike state. All displayed the same "body language," regardless of age, gender, or social status. They were perfectly calm, almost motionless unless instructed to move, with faces whose expressions can best be described as placid, perhaps even serene. This demeanor did not change when they were stabbed, sliced, or punctured during a treatment procedure, or sat seemingly uninvolved during a disobsession, as long as they were in fact participating in the therapeutic ritual interacting as a patient or an observer. My guess was that it was during the orientation sessions, when the patients and those accompanying them quietly sat through the seemingly endless, repetitive invocations to the spirits and testimonials by those previously healed, that so many inadvertently went into a hypnotic or altered state of consciousness.

All the other Kardecist-Spiritists with whom I raised the subject echoed the denials of Dr. Fritz. I had no reason to believe they'd collectively engaged in deliberate concealment. But I was now convinced, along with the practitioners of hypnosis and hypnotherapy who'd seen the videos, that patients were anesthetized through something like a hypnotic induction process, with results equivalent to hypnotism. This appeared also to be true for those being disobssessed. Furthermore, the reports of little or no pain in the hours and days following surgery by those operated on sounded very much like the effects of powerful posthypnotic suggestion.

Did the patients "go under" in a way similar to those at an entertainment hypnotist's performance? While none in such an audience can be hypnotized against his or her will, many quickly enter into at least some level of trance without consciously being aware of it or seeking to do so. The brief and subtle interactions between the audience and the hypnotist on stage are produced by well-established techniques.

When "mesmerized" in this way, subjects uncritically accept information from the hypnotist about what to perceive or remember and how to behave both during and after being "entranced." They may at times seem like spontaneous sleepwalkers, but unlike true sleepwalkers, their brain waves remain those of waking individuals. Anyone who is especially responsive will see, hear, feel, smell, and taste in accordance with the suggestions given, even when they contradict objective reality—often a source of amusement for onlookers. Clearly, the volunteer performer's consciousness has been altered, although no truly unacceptable command will be followed.

Edson/Fritz and others engaged in Spiritist activities denied any such practice. I watched carefully. I never saw him, or any of the other healer-mediums I observed, displaying what I now knew to be the hypnotist's craft. Besides, to block acute pain, consciousness would have to be altered far more than is necessary to merely entertain an audience.

I pressed Dr. Fritz with additional questions. Why, I asked, was it necessary to perform surgeries? Why cut into patients when all healing, as I had learned after my experiences in Porto Alegre, Palmelo, Campo Grande, Rio de Janeiro, and elsewhere in the country, was done by spirits who had no need to use material means but instead could rely on the "more advanced" spiritual techniques developed in the other, or spirit, world? Why take the risk of performing invasive procedures that might expose patients to possible physical dangers that were not necessary? Moreover, why do the surgeries in public places where they attract attention, such as from the Brazilian medical establishment, who invariably react by calling in the legal authorities?

"You are right," Edson/Fritz growled at me, making explicit something he might have preferred not to have said. Cutting really is not necessary. It is done, he added with studied emphasis, "only to catch people's attention."

"Catch their attention," I muttered, restraining my sense of shock. "But why?" I persisted. "Why cut people when you do not have to?"

"Because people do not believe," was his pointed reply. "They must be shown. And when they are," he continued with satisfaction, "they will have no choice but to accept the truth."

What Fritz meant by this, as he elaborated on other occasions during taped interviews given to me in private, was that people generally do not accept the basic "truths" of Spiritism and so do not adopt its teachings and practices. When they observe, or better yet *experience,* a Spiritist surgery, it definitely catches their attention, especially when patients are cut and neither antisepsis nor anesthesia is used. Moreover, those operated on usually experience little or no pain and recover without complications. This startling fact, he reasoned aloud, would force people to think and to ask how what they have experienced or witnessed could be explained? The point was expressed on an engraved plaque prominently displayed at a center where another healer-medium I visited treated patients. It read: "For the believer, no explanation is necessary. For the nonbeliever, no explanation is possible."

The events, Dr. Fritz continued, defied people's conventional frames of comprehension, those that formed their commonsense understandings. The surgeries were anomalies that could not be accounted for by the paradigms on which modern scientific medicine is based. Unable to find any other explanation, Dr. Fritz reasoned, the patients, those who accompany them, and the observers became receptive to the Spiritist view that what they had experienced was performed by disincarnate beings from a world whose existence they did not ordinarily acknowledge. In brief, the surgeries, before which patients and those accompanying them were exposed to lengthy lectures and personal testimonials (delivered in a stylized monotone) that made explicit Spiritist belief and cosmology, were part of a program of conversion and indoctrination. In addition to helping the sick, in the Brazilian elaboration of what Kardec had first proposed, Brazilian Spiritists like José Carlos, Edson, Mauricio, Antonio, Fernando, and Drs. Lacerda and Hervé had transformed their ritual practices into dramatic healing sessions in an intentional effort to "hook" both the patients and the observing public so as to convert them to Spiritist beliefs.

Spiritists, I soon realized, were not the only group in Brazil with a distinctive view of the world and its own cosmology that used unconventional religious rituals to heal the sick, hoping in the process to attract converts. Over the next decade, I learned that therapeutic interventions that could not be explained by the conventional sciences that had come to provide the bases for our commonsense understandings of illness and healing were at the core of each group's proselytizing, and that all groups were in vigorous competition with each other for new converts.

PART II

HEALING BY THE SPIRITS IN OTHER BRAZILIAN POPULAR RELIGIONS

CHAPTER 8

RELIGION AND RELIGIOUS DIVERSITY IN BRAZILIAN HISTORY

In 1500, when a Portuguese fleet under the command of Pedro Álvares Cabral laid anchor at Porto Seguro in what is now the Bay of Bahia, Europeans officially "discovered" Brazil. Cabral disembarked, planted the flag, and claimed the territory in the name of the Crown. Then he and his armada proceeded on to the Orient, their original destination. The objective of the voyage was to secure trading arrangements for the valuable commercial goods that Vasco da Gama had reported finding there after his historic voyage around the Cape of Good Hope the year before.

Six years earlier, two years after Columbus first arrived in the New World, Pope Alexander VI had divided the world as he knew it, ceding dominion over one half to Portugal and the other half to Spain in what has come to be known as the Treaty of Tordesilhas. Even before the document was signed, Portugal requested that the line of demarcation be moved westward to 200 leagues from the Cape Verde Islands. When Spain agreed, the undiscovered lands of Brazil became part of Portugal's overseas domain.

The first fifty years of the sixteenth century was a period of significant religious turmoil in Europe. Although still predominant, the Roman Catholic Church was in shambles. Scandals marked the short tenures of each of the seven popes who occupied the Vatican and reigned an average of only seven years each.

Martin Luther tacked his ninety-five theses on the door of Wittenberg Church seventeen years into the century, culminating in agitation for religious reform that began with the efforts of men like John Wycliffe in England and John Huss in Czechoslovakia. The Reformation and the schism in Christianity led to the establishment of independent Protestant churches. The resulting religious conflict, violence, and warfare were to plague Europe and the world for centuries to come.

The papal decree of 1494 may be seen as part of the Vatican's response to the growing pressure that was to result in the Reformation. Spain and Portugal, the two most powerful kingdoms in Europe, both ardently Catholic, were given, and accepted, responsibility to bring the "true faith" to those throughout the world who had not yet been converted. Ignatius of Loyola founded the Society of Jesus in 1540, the Inquisition was established two years later, and the Council of Trent was held in 1545. These three instruments of the Counter-Reformation were the basis of the church's response to what it viewed as the Protestant heresy.

The Portuguese Crown and its million or so subjects focused their limited resources on the lucrative Asian trade rather than on the lands of the Southern Cross, as Brazil was then called, where little of commercial value was to be found. Portugal sent missionaries to Brazil, with the task of converting the aborigines; the Jesuits arrived to lead the effort in 1549.

Shortly after mid-century, King John III, trying to protect the colony from other (read Protestant) Europeans who coveted it, delineated twelve vast tracts of land, starting on the Atlantic coast and extending inland as far as the never-actually-measured Tordesilhas line. He granted the lands to members of the Portuguese nobility, with the expectation that they would occupy them. The only two recipients who actually took possession mimicked the successful Portuguese settlements in the Atlantic islands, where sugarcane was grown. Sugar, raised with slave labor, had created great wealth since the early fifteenth century. Some two thousand islanders were among the settlers who came to the northeast coast to colonize and carve out plantations. With the Iberian newcomers came slaves, captured on the African mainland and pressed into service to produce the crop. The Portuguese already had decided that the New World natives, primarily hunters and gatherers who wandered through the forests, made poor sedentary agricultural workers. Almost immediately, Brazilian sugar brought to landowners, merchants, and the Crown a wealth that was comparable to that earned by trade in the Orient.

The Portuguese pattern of colonization was for men to come alone and to send for spouses later. The males did not remain celibate but mated with native women and female slaves, producing a mixed population that was to become characteristic of the society. As the men were establishing the economic and political order of the colony as an extension of Europe, women, who knew only Amerindian or African cultural practices, were shaping local domestic life. As a result, there was a syncretic mixing of many aspects of what was to develop into a national culture.

Brazil, officially Roman Catholic, was organized formally into parishes, where local churches were built. Its settlers practiced a pre-Reformation form of the religion that focused on processions, making vows to the saints, and pilgrimages to shrines rather than on what the official church was doing to combat the growing Protestant heresy. Since there were never enough priests in Brazil to do more than present the catechism to slaves, say occasional masses, and perform baptisms, weddings, and funerals, Brazilians were little influenced by the clergy.

In daily life on the far-flung, sparsely settled, isolated sugar estates, the owners and their managers were interested primarily in how much the slaves produced. Little time or energy was spent on what the slaves or their mixed-blood children did in private. Nor were owners and managers concerned that slaves were able to maintain and transmit to succeeding generations components of their African worlds. Beliefs and practices of their homelands were often mixed with elements of "popular" Catholicism. Deities—the orixás, for example—were called by both African and Catholic saint names. In this way aspects of African sacred worlds were kept alive in Brazil and syncretized with medieval European practices, although these same practices were being discarded most other places in the Roman Catholic world.

By the beginning of the seventeenth century, the population of Brazil was estimated at 100,000—30,000 of them European. A century later it had grown to 300,000, still one-third European. By then, groups of Portuguese who had settled in and around what is now São Paulo, accompanied by their native mates and followers, had discovered diamonds and gold in the backlands beyond the coastal mountains (pushing the Tordesilhas line ever westward as they trekked into the interior). This led, as Furtado (1963:80) observed, to a "spontaneous migratory flow [of colonists from Portugal] for the first time." Between 300,000 and 500,000 people—mostly men—from the interior provinces of Portugal had arrived before the precious minerals ran out at the end of the century. Of lower socioeconomic status than the earlier colonists, they too adopted the practice of using the labor of African slaves to dig, pan, and clean the precious stones and minerals from the soil. As in the sugar-producing northeast, the men here mated with slave women; a biologically mixed population came to characterize the new region called Minas Gerais, "the general mines." As the men set out Lusitanian patterns of political and economic organization, their African mates and slave dependents were left to organize once more most aspects of domestic life. By 1800 the colonial population had reached 3.25 million, consisting of more than a million African slaves, an unknown number of racially mixed people, and the remainder Europeans.

The third economic boom—coffee production—opened yet another part of the westward-expanding country.[18] The pattern of European emigrants using imported African captives to produce wealth and creating a biologically mixed population, with men establishing European-oriented political and economic orders and dependent minority women being responsible for domestic life, was repeated. The combination of official Catholicism and de facto African American religious syncretism also was replicated.

In the first decade of the nineteenth century, the Portuguese court was forced to move across the Atlantic Ocean to Rio de Janeiro to escape Napoleon's advancing armies. The New World city became the capital of the empire. After Napoleon was defeated, instead of returning home, the heir to the Portuguese Crown decided to remain in Brazil. Declaring Brazil independent in 1822, he assumed the title emperor.

In 1888, in another decree, the second emperor's daughter officially abolished slavery. Meanwhile, large numbers of Europeans were pouring into Brazil, just as they were into the United States, Argentina, and other parts of the Americas. They brought customs and traditions that emerged in the twentieth century as a regionally and ethnically diverse national culture, gradually reorganized away from Portuguese institutional patterns.

Until Brazil became a republic in a bloodless coup in 1889, Roman Catholicism remained the official religion. Thereafter, as the nation experienced a variety of governments and constitutions, Brazilians were free to choose their religion. Although they began as nominally Roman Catholic, and that remains mostly true today, they had many alternatives to the official Catholic Church, including a popular variant that focused on the saints, processions, and pilgrimages. In addition, there was a range of localized, African-derived, syncretic belief systems practiced in *terreiros*, places of worship that varied from region to region.

After two earlier failures, Protestantism arrived in Brazil, now carried by emigrants from Europe and missionaries, first from England and then from the United States. Numerous Protestant denominations, aiming to attract followers from the Catholic fold, were quickly added to the growing religious mix.

The original philosophical thinking of Allan Kardec was fashioned to take religious form and offered to the public at Spiritist centers. His beliefs, syncretized with a diffuse set of African practices, as we shall see in chapter 11, gave birth to Umbanda. Emigrants from Japan and elsewhere in Asia added other religious forms to expand the range of alternatives available to the 18 million Brazilians free to choose their religion as the twentieth century opened.

As elsewhere in the world, religions mobilized to compete with each other for the hearts and minds of the populace. In contrast with the spread of faiths in most places, Brazilian religions offered healing, combined to a lesser degree with relief from the practical problems of daily life, as well as words and sentiments promising a better future in this world and the next.

As the nation urbanized, industrialized, modernized, and even globalized in the second half of the century, the number of inhabitants increased tenfold, growing to 180 million by 2000. As a result of these transformations potential converts had an ever-growing number of problems. Each religion offered its own version of the supernatural to assist with them. Religious healers volunteered to provide assistance with a range of human afflictions, only some of which now involved health care or had a medical diagnosis.

The chapters in this section examine how different religions provide help in exchange for membership. The resulting social patterns are referred to as a religious marketplace. Each faith is presented as a provider offering a product to a population of consumers making choices among them. The overarching rule, taken from the popular Catholic tradition, is of a consumer making a purchase, an offer of exchange to the supernatural that is conditional. Only if the consumer is satisfied—that is, cured or otherwise aided—is he or she committed to make payment. That payment involves affiliating with the community, accepting its teachings, and performing its rituals. In this way, Brazilians move from one religion to another as they seek relief for existing and ever-increasing new infirmities. A single individual may convert and become a member of a series of diverse and competing religions over the course of a lifetime. Members of the same household may worship in different places.

Why Brazilian religions came to choose to offer healing or other forms of help by their supernatural(s) as the primary tools in their competition for converts has no definitive answer as yet. Certainly, the wealth produced by the society has been inequitably distributed to the population ever since the Portuguese took possession of the New World territory. Poverty abounds and has been exacerbated with modernization and globalization. But Brazil is not the only nation characterized by massive poverty, with a skewed and unjust distribution of its wealth. Numbers of illnesses known to afflict the poor primarily are not significantly higher for Brazil than other places. So why have religious groups there come to focus on healing?

An interesting series of writings by Alfred W. Crosby ([1986], 1993, 1972) proposes the thesis that when the Europeans conquered and colonized much of the world in the period following Columbus, as they decimated and replaced populations, they also brought with them fauna and flora, micro and macro, and ways of interacting with them that transformed local ecologies.

For millions of years, divergent species had adapted to a variety of local environments that were continuously changing in response to series of major geological transformations of the landscape. The introduction of people and their biota from across the oceans millenniums later had unintended consequences that contributed inadvertently to the European takeover of much of the planet (see Diamond 1997).

Crosby used the concept of Neo-Europe to refer to the ecological systems brought by Europeans that took hold in so many parts of the world. Most of these places, he observes, were in temperate zones. In the tropics, Europeans generally encountered densely inhabited human settlements, each with its own respective fauna, flora, and micro-universes that they could not replace.[19] Brazil was the only Neo-Europe to be established on a large landmass in the tropics.

Could it be that for the past several centuries—a tiny period for species adapted to temperate zones to readapt to the tropics—European emigrants and their African servants, who brought their own array of life-forms, have been involved in adapting to a new environmental setting? Is it possible that many of the aches and pains reported by this ever more biologically mixed and growing population, which seem to defy medical classification and are usually dismissed as psychosomatic, are a manifestation of this adaptive process? Could recognition of these many unexplained cases of human unease, added to incidences of illness associated with poverty, have brought the leaders of religious groups in Brazil to focus their competitive quest for converts on healing? The data to answer these questions are not yet available. But raising them may contribute to future research and add to our understanding of the complexities of culture, biology, and, more specifically for our purposes, religion, medicine, and healing.

We do know that treating human affliction is the product that religious groups in Brazil offer prospective consumers in the religious marketplace. The remaining chapters in this section examine some of the other groups that provide healing or other forms of assistance by their supernatural(s) in exchange for affiliation. The final chapter elaborates on how individuals make decisions and choices to navigate in the marketplace as they seek help with their many and varied personal problems.

CHAPTER 9

PILGRIMAGE AND HEALING IN "POPULAR" CATHOLICISM

The exemplar adopted in modified or syncretized form by all of Brazil's religious groups in their efforts to attract followers in a country in which Roman Catholicism was once the official religion is Catholicism—not as presented by the official church in Rome and its appointees in Brazil, but in the way it was practiced when first brought to the Western Hemisphere by the early colonists and settlers from the Iberian Peninsula. It is to this pre-Reformation Catholicism—characterized by processions, vows to the saints, and pilgrimages to shrines taking place outside the church edifice—that I turn first.

I had an opportunity to see how it works in Brazil in the fall of 1981. Drs. Antonio Mourão Cavalcante and Adalberto Barreto, two young friends I'd met shortly after my original encounter with José Carlos (both Brazilian-trained psychiatrists recently returned from Europe, where they had been completing doctoral degrees in anthropology), took me to the annual Festa de São Francisco (St. Francis of Assisi Festival) in Canindé, a small municipality in the arid backlands of the state of Ceará, that was the home of a basilica dedicated to the Italian saint. In this part of the world, people called him São Francisco das Chagas (St. Francis of the Wounds), ostensibly to differentiate him from the Old World version and to make him their own. I was to visit Canindé frequently over the next decade, to participate in conferences on popular religion that my colleagues and I organized in cooperation with the Franciscan brothers and to study the *romeiros*, or pilgrims, who came by the millions to make their *promessas*, or vows, to the saint at the annual *festa*. What follows is a summary of the relationship between pilgrimage and healing as told through the stories of some of the participants.

When the driver suddenly applied the brakes to the rickety old truck while making the sharp turn onto the traffic-congested road marked "Canindé," Maria da Fatima Batista braced herself on the backless bench she had occupied for much of the previous four days. She was almost there. Her dream was about to be realized.

It had all begun some five years earlier, when Fatima fell from a cart in the fields where she toiled as an agricultural worker. She had hurt her leg. After several weeks of medical treatment, the swelling was still there and the pain even worse. Unable to do her job, she even had difficulty caring for her home, her spouse, and their children.

This thirty-year-old laborer from the small municipality of Regeneração, in the interior of the northeastern Brazilian state of Piauí, was not a religious person, although she had been raised Catholic and confirmed in her youth. It had been many years since Fatima had entered a church or even thought about the world of the supernatural. Now, desperate, she turned to St. Francis, the saint she had heard so much about. With as much fervor as she could muster, she addressed the holy being. Fatima concentrated, focusing her attention completely on the saint whose help she was requesting, promising aloud in a soft and deferential voice that if she received it, she would visit his shrine on the anniversary of his birth and light candles, attend mass, take confession, walk the stations of the cross, and dress in a *mortalha*, a brown habit similar to the one he wore. Fatima vowed, as an additional expression of her lowliness, dependence, and humility in the face of this powerful heavenly figure, that if healed she would cut off her beautiful and much-admired waist-length black hair at the shrine in Canindé.

In the weeks to follow, her leg improved. She gradually resumed her normal activities, even returning to work at the end of the month. Soon thereafter, the pain disappeared completely.

When Fatima told her cousin what had happened, and of her vow and subsequent "miraculous" recovery, Maria Laura offered to accompany her when she went to Canindé. Laura's own visit there had been, in her words, "the high point of my life." Returning, although requiring great sacrifice, would give her untold pleasure. Laura informed her cousin that Sr. Pedro, who freighted goods in the area, carried passengers to Canindé for the festival. She volunteered to find out how much he charged and to estimate how much money they would need for food and other supplies during the ten-day trip. Realizing immediately that they had nowhere near the amount of money necessary, the women knew that St. Francis would understand the delay and wait patiently to receive his due. Four years later, after saving small amounts from their wages periodically and selling several of the animals their families raised, they had accumulated sufficient money. Six months before the festival, they contacted Sr. Pedro and reserved two places on his *pau-de-arara* ("parrot's perch"), as such trucks are called.

The night before leaving, joined by family and friends who reminisced of their own experiences, the cousins carefully packed their food, a small stove, two hammocks, clothes, and other necessities, including a small wooden leg that Fatima's spouse had carved as a votive offering. Added to their belongings were gifts to be deposited at the shrine from friends unable to make the trip themselves. Arriving at the designated place by mule cart before dawn, the cousins met the truck and were on their way.

For the next four days, Fatima, Laura, and the other faithful bounced uncomfortably across the dry, barren moonscape known as the *sertão*, a semidesert the size of France and Spain. There had been no rain that year, or the previous one, and the riverbeds were dry. The plants that managed to sprout had withered quickly due to the lack of water; livestock carcasses were strewn along the roadside. The driver stopped the truck only when necessary, always at deserted roadsides, so the passengers could prepare and eat meals, relieve themselves, rest in the late afternoon heat, and sleep at night. Four flat tires further complicated the journey and delayed their arrival at the shrine.

Although Fatima was not consciously aware of it, she had become part of a tradition that stretched back well over two millennia. A pilgrimage in Christian tradition is a visit to the shrine of a saint, where a powerful and mystical religious intensity is believed to be present. The practice has its roots in both the Greco-Roman and Hebrew traditions. Visiting sacred places did not become an important part of religious worship until after Constantine's conversion in the fourth century, when Christianity became the religion of the Roman Empire (Carroll 2001). From then on, when the faith was carried to other parts of the world, pilgrimage to the shrines of saints was central to the complex of beliefs and practices to which the pagan peoples of northern and eastern Europe, Asia, and eventually the New World were (often forcibly) exposed.

The earliest Christian saints were martyrs who gave their lives for their faith. After Constantine, a new model of sainthood emerged: members of local communities would decide that one of their more admired fellows, who had healed or performed other acts of wonder in life, had done so because God had so ordained it and was working his miracles through that person. When the individual died, those familiar with the events attributed to the deceased would flock to the grave and request in death what had been given so freely in life. When it was received, a shrine was placed at the tomb; stories would circulate far and wide about the extraordinary events taking place there. On hearing the tales, others in need of help would visit the tomb. In time the shrine would become a holy place of worship.[20]

Although the importance of the cult of the saints and pilgrimage declined in religious life after the Reformation, even among Catholics, both remained vital elements practiced by the inhabitants of the Iberian Peninsula. When, in the late fifteenth and sixteenth centuries, the Portuguese embarked on the conquest and colonization of their part of the Western Hemisphere, they brought the cult of the saints and pilgrimage as central features of their Christianity.

Going on pilgrimage is not an independent activity but rather an aspect of the cult of the saints (Brown 1981). "Reborn" and elevated to everlasting life in heaven by an all-powerful creator God, believed to have control over all aspects of the universe, including the destinies of those on earth, saints are considered "friends of God," able to act as intermediaries with him on behalf of supplicants on earth. As

Wilson (1983:23) phrases the position proclaimed in official church theology, saints "might be seen as advocates pleading causes before a stern judge, as mediators, as go-betweens, as intriguers or wire-pullers, at the court of Heaven."

The faithful may invoke a saint's help with material as well as spiritual problems through prayer and petition. This supernatural intervention in our world is referred to as a miracle. Miracles, as Augustine of Hippo was so influential in maintaining, "were signs of God's power and proof of the sanctity of those in whose name they were wrought" (Woodward 1990:62).

"The relationship between a saint and a devotee in Brazil," as Queiroz (1973:86) observes, "is one of reciprocity, or better of *dou ut des:* I give to receive something in exchange." For it to work, the petitioner must know what the saint likes and dislikes, how he wishes to be treated, and his ritual preferences. The petitioner must include these preferences in his or her vow. Furthermore, the petition must be made in a way that will entice the saint to accept the bargain. Vows are made conditionally. They do not have to be fulfilled (discharged) unless and until the petitioner obtains what has been requested. Christian, particularly Catholic, pilgrimage is part of the cult of the saints and what since the Reformation (and Counter-Reformation) has been called "popular"—as opposed to official—Catholicism.

Representatives of the Portuguese Crown and the church brought Christianity to the territory that was to become Brazil when the New World colony was occupied. It was the colony's official religion until Brazil became a republic at the end of the nineteenth century (1889), some six and a half decades after national independence had been attained in 1822. Christian practice, institutionalization, and diffusion, as Freyre (1964) and others (e.g., Azzi 1978) have reminded us, were mostly a private matter. Many founders of the great family houses established around the production of sugarcane, the mining of gold and diamonds, and other economic boom activities had their own domestic shrines and chapels. Shrines also were built in out-of-the-way places, mostly in gratitude to a specific saint or the Virgin for some good fortune obtained there, believed to have been the result of an intercession and a response to prayer.

Priests, always in short supply in Brazil, were brought in when available to say masses, perform baptisms, weddings, and funerals, and to teach catechism to slaves and other dependents, but most of the "religious" activity practiced throughout Brazilian history was a personal dynamic between a "believer" and a saint at a private shrine. As Bastide (1951:346) observed some time ago, popular religious worship in Brazil is turned more toward the saints and the Virgin than God.

The saints venerated during the early years of the colonial period were those brought from the Old World and listed in the official church calendar. The pau-de-arara carrying Maria da Fatima and her fellow pilgrims went to the shrine of one of these saints. The shrine is said to have been founded in the late eighteen century by Francisco Xavier de Madeiros, a Portuguese sergeant major traveling in the region who, for reasons not reported, wished to build a chapel on the banks of the Canindé River in honor of the saint after whom he had been named.[21]

When construction was delayed due to one of the periodic droughts that plague this part of the country, a statue of the saint was brought to the site. Reports began to circulate about the sick and injured recovering "miraculously." People from surrounding neighborhoods started visiting the statue. Those "blessed" left gifts that were used to complete the first church. Donations made over the years were applied to build numerous additions.

Today a large basilica stands where Madeiros first planned his church. Public and commercial buildings are located to the north of it, across from the *praça*, or square. The streets spread out in all directions, with the more substantial homes of prosperous merchants and landowners located closest to the basilica, as they are in all small towns in the Brazilian interior, and the poorer ones stretching up an incline to the urban periphery, where tire repair shops, Afro-Brazilian religious centers, brothels, and other marginal commercial establishments can be found. The basilica, at the center, contains the holy activities. Just beyond it, along the river, is the Grotto of Nossa Senhora de Lourdes. It is here where pilgrims go to wash, drink the water, and fill receptacles for friends and relatives unable to make the trip. Water from the grotto is believed to have miraculous curing properties (Cavalcante 1987:6).

Located beyond the basilica is an area that houses a museum and a zoological garden owned and operated by the Franciscan brothers. Further on is a zone of religious commerce; beyond that one finds prepared foods, beverages (including alcohol), and many manufactured items. Next come games of chance, pool, and an amusement park with a huge Ferris wheel, other rides, and various forms of entertainment. Finally, at the outskirts, there are bars, dance halls, and *vai quem quer* (go whoever wishes), as the local houses of prostitution are picturesquely called.

Preparations for the influx of pilgrims begin some six weeks before the official mass that opens the annual festival on September 24. The Franciscan brothers make ready the simple shelters called *abrigos* that will house those visitors unable to afford space in hotels and private dwellings. They will set up and clean makeshift lavatories, places to bathe, and cooking facilities. Many residents who have family homes in the nearby rural hinterland, or relatives with whom they can stay, rent their primary houses to more affluent pilgrims. The merchants prepare their shops to make room for crosses; rosaries; pictures; statues of St. Francis, the Virgin, and other saints; foods; beverages; clothing; plastic toys; and other commercial items. Townspeople and residents of neighboring municipalities seeking to earn extra money set up stalls and booths, most often using poles, scraps of wood, and old pieces of cardboard brought in by truck from Fortaleza, the state capital and main commercial center some 90 kilometers distant. Those who live in or near Canindé depend on what they earn during the festival to sustain them throughout the year. Approximately one million people visit Canindé and its shrine annually, most during the ten days of the celebration at the end of September and the beginning of October.

When the vehicle from Regeneração turned off the pothole-filled, weather-beaten road on which it had crossed the backlands onto the new paved highway that led into Canindé, it joined with many other paus-de-arara bringing pilgrims from all over the Brazilian northeast. The slow-moving lanes also contained buses rented especially for the occasion, private automobiles, and a number of horses and horse-drawn carriages. Some pilgrims came from great distances on bicycles; others came on foot.

Most of the visitors were from Ceará, while others came from neighboring states in northeastern Brazil. Pilgrims also came from as far away as São Paulo, Rio de Janeiro, and even Europe and North America.

Many of the travelers, like Maria da Fatima and her cousin, were agricultural laborers, domestic servants, or unemployed. One-third of some two thousand pilgrims interviewed in the mid-1980s reported having neither land nor homes of their own but living on properties that belonged to large estates, to which they paid a share of what they grew. Half reported migrating periodically, hoping to find better living conditions (Barreto 1986:3). The number of men and women were approximately equal, and although many of the pilgrims were poor, as are the vast majority of Brazilians, all social classes and racial and ethnic categories were represented in Canindé.

The truck carrying Maria da Fatima stopped at one of the abrigos located not far from the basilica. Finding space available there, the occupants strung their hammocks on hooks and stored the food, clothing, and various items they had brought with them. Then, although it was late in the day and they had not eaten since before noon, the two women left, walking along the street that led to the basilica. A *lambe lambe* (photographer) was taking Polaroid snapshots. Fatima waited in line to have herself photographed wearing the brown habit of St. Francis, holding votive offerings, and standing next to a life-sized cardboard cutout of the saint. A half hour later, the two were again on their way to the basilica and the Casa dos Milagres, a large room adorned with thousands of pictures of pilgrims and the material representations of their "miracles." Fatima placed one copy of the Polaroid snapshot on the wall. The other she would keep and put next to her bed at home. The next part of her vow was completed when she walked across the room to deposit her ex-voto. A huge receptacle was overflowing with thousands of crudely fashioned votives made mostly of balsa wood, local bamboo, clay, and cloth. Seen also were beautifully carved pieces made of fine wood, probably commissioned by people of means and made by professional craftsmen. The pile was so high that Fatima had to climb a ladder and stretch to get her ex-voto to the top of the stack.

Fatima and Laura went next to a small room where a beautician stood shearing a woman's hair. The woman, Clarice Magalhães de Sousa, also wearing a brown habit that masked her middle-class status, had traveled by bus with her husband, a bank lawyer, from the capital of the state of Rio Grande do Norte, several hundred miles away. For their stay in Canindé, the Sousas rented a room with bed and a bath. They took their meals in restaurants, where they ate eggs with their coffee for breakfast and meat and vegetables with rice and beans for lunch and dinner.

Dona Clarice had been diagnosed some years previously with breast cancer. Before undertaking the surgery and radiation treatment prescribed by her doctor, she had prayed to St. Francis, promising him that if he cured her she would not only make the pilgrimage to Canindé, attend mass, take confession, and light candles at his shrine but also cut off her shoulder-length hair. Certainly, the educated and sophisticated Sousas knew that her recovery could be attributed to modern medical science. But could it not also have been intercession by the saint? Like so many others, Dona Clarice had made a bargain with St. Francis before undertaking medical treatment. She had compensated her doctors as soon as she received their bill. Now she was paying what she owed to the saint.

Like Dona Clarice, most Brazilians, as we have seen with the Kardecist-Spiritists, seek doctors or other healers when they are hurt or take sick, but this does not stop them from also praying to saints or seeking help from other supernatural beings. They acknowledge that surgery and medications provided by trained medical practitioners work, but more so when complemented by supernatural assistance. Many, like Fatima, Laura, and patients of José Carlos, Edson, Antonio, and Mauricio, also believe that supernatural intervention on its own can help them.

Angela, a young lady from the state of Paraíba, waited anxiously for the beautician to finish with Dona Clarice. She had sat in the same chair the year before but had been unable to fulfill her vow at that time because she was "too vain" to face life without her beautiful hair. The high-strung, nervous woman had suffered from severe headaches, and although a doctor had prescribed medicine, the pains had worsened. She began to pray to St. Francis. When the symptoms abated, she knew a pilgrimage had to be made to discharge her obligations. Angela returned to Canindé, this time prepared to give the saint his due.

"Do you think that St. Francis will forgive you?" we asked her.

"Yes he will," she responded, "because he has forgiven more than this. I have faith, I believe that he will."

When Fatima's turn came, feelings of sadness and gratitude filled her. Certainly, she would miss her beautiful hair, but she felt virtuous about losing it for such a special reason. Fatima took the bag in which the cuttings of her hair were placed. Like Dona Clarice and Angela before her, she returned to the Casa dos Milagres to put it on top of the heap of votive offerings. Having completed this very personal and emotional part of her vow, Fatima joined her cousin. They returned to the abrigo to start a fire on which they would cook the rice and beans that would be their dinner. Several hours later, after cleaning up and storing their belongings, exhilarated but exhausted, they climbed into their hammocks and tried to sleep.

At dawn, when Fatima and Laura joined a long line of pilgrims waiting for the lavatories and bathing facilities, the city and the festival were already bursting with activities. Their breakfast, which consisted solely of coffee laced with ample sugar, was prepared as hastily as possible. Then they were off to the basilica once again. As they entered the courtyard on their way to the church office where they would learn the schedule of masses and confessions, they came upon Pedro, a young man from Fortaleza who had made the trip to Canindé on his bicycle. He was circling the church on his knees. His mother had been sick. "It was her leg," he said, "the left one." She had gone to the doctor and had almost lost the limb. They had had to graft parts from other places on her body to make the necessary repairs. She was in a cast for four months. "But now she is well, thanks to God and St. Francis." Pedro had prayed to the saint on her behalf, promising that if she recovered, he would make the pilgrimage and walk around the courtyard on his knees, not once but twice. He was now completing his second turn. Although it was difficult and he was uncomfortable and sore, he was pleased that he had fulfilled his debt to the saint. He could return home satisfied and at peace.

At the small church office, a volunteer provided the women with the schedule of masses. When Fatima revealed that it had been more than ten years since she had last been to church, she was told that she would have to attend a preparation class before entering the confessional booth. Since the session was about to begin, the women hurried to the designated room. Forty-five minutes later, they took their places in a line that stretched the length of the basilica to wait their turn at the confessional. Afterward they walked back to the abrigo to prepare, cook, and eat the rice and beans that would be their lunch. Several hours later they hurried to the basilica again, this time to attend mass. Joining other devotees afterward, they walked the stations of the cross, the symbolic representation of the route taken by Jesus through Jerusalem to Calvary.

When Fatima picked up a stone to place on her head to increase the penance, she accidentally bumped into Sergio, a young man reaching for a rock at the same time. He had made the trip on foot from Fortaleza, where he attended university. After twice failing the *vestibular,* a standardized examination that all Brazilian students must pass to gain admission to university, he made a vow to St. Francis before attempting the test for a third time. Now a freshman studying computer science, he was fulfilling his debt to the saint for the help he had received in surmounting the obstacle. As he, Fatima, and a score of others proceeded solemnly along the path, changing rocks at each station, the temperature exceeded 90°F under a blazing sun. The women stopped to drink a cup of water, which they purchased from a girl sitting on the roadside with a bucket she had filled at a standpipe. Next they went to the museum to see some of the exquisite jewels and garments used in church services by the Franciscan brothers.

The two pilgrims wandered together through the stalls. They were tempted by both religious and secular items, few of which they could afford. Each did purchase one or two gifts commissioned by friends and relatives and some small souvenirs for their families. By this time they were exhausted. They returned to the abrigo to begin preparations for the evening meal. After cooking and eating more rice and beans, they set out for the secular festival. As women traveling alone, they rejected visiting the bars and dancing establishments frequented by men. They concentrated on games of chance for their entertainment. At about 9:00 p.m., when they returned to the abrigo, they were too excited to go to bed and instead sat for several hours talking and sharing with each other the joy they were experiencing. Each slept very little that night.

The following morning, after several long and tedious hours devoted to the same daily activities, the two women went to the grotto, where they washed themselves in its curative waters. They drank and filled plastic containers, which they would take back to Regeneração for friends and relatives.

Their next destination was the Franciscan monastery, where they patiently stood with hundreds of others in the courtyard to observe and talk to a life-sized statue of the saint. When her turn came, after more than an hour of waiting, Fatima, like each of the others before her, quietly but intensely conversed aloud with the saint. She thanked him, commenting to the statute about very personal matters and petitioning help with other problems. Afterward, Laura excitedly led her into a small room near the entryway to the monastery. A group of pilgrims stood there, trying to peek through the door of an inner room. A rumor was circulating that St. Francis was inside, alive, and that in fact he had never died. The Franciscans were keeping him there, unwilling to share him with the pilgrims. When nothing further happened, the women concluded the report to be untrue.

Returning to the abrigo, they began again the lengthy task of preparing their rice and beans. After a short rest, they visited the zoological gardens, where they spent the next few hours looking at the animals, most of which they had never seen before. They giggled as they went from cage to cage, commenting on the magnificent colors of some of the birds and laughing at the strange postures assumed by other animals. Like most visitors, their favorites were the monkeys, in front of whose cage they stood enthralled. Soon it was time to return to the abrigo, collect their belongings, and place them aboard the waiting truck. By late afternoon they were on the road again, headed for Regeneração. During the next four days, as they bounced uncomfortably across the back roads of the sertão on the crowded truck, the women repeated aloud to each other, perhaps in a rehearsal of what they would tell their loved ones when they arrived home, the details of, and their emotions about, the experience they had shared.

Research conducted in the late 1950s found that 80 percent of the visitors to the shrine of St. Francis in Canindé were there because they claimed to have been healed (Hooneart 1987:5). Yet pilgrims, like the patients of Kardecist healer-mediums, rarely use such terms as *illness* or *disease*. Instead they speak of pains in the back, leg, or head, or the inability to walk. Their assumption is that God has caused their suffering to punish them for the commission of a sin. The saint's intercession leads to the removal of the cause of their pain. Hence they are "cured."

In another study, conducted over a five-year period between 1984 and 1988, Barreto and his students in the Department of Social Medicine at the Federal University of Ceará collected, examined, and classified more than 80,000 ex-votos. More than 86 percent of

(Upper left) São Francisco de Chagas in Canindé. (Upper right) Pilgrims dressed in "mortalha" worn by St. Francis. (Middle) Votive offerings. (Lower left) Woman offering her hair as a votive offering. (Lower right) Hair of pilgrim being cut in fulfillment of her vow.

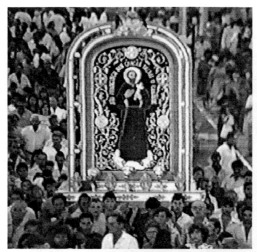
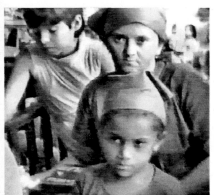
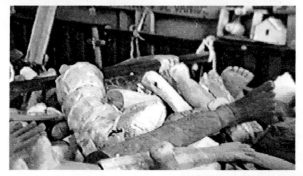
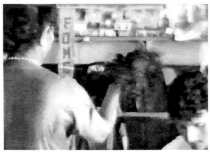
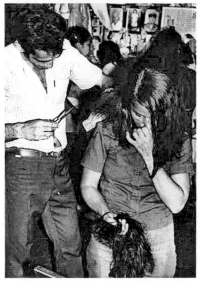

them represented parts of the body that the saint was believed to have healed. Of these, almost 5,000 showed wounds, cuts, or other openings in the skin; 2,350 showed protuberances indicating edemas or growths; 1,400 represented disfigurements of the skin or other dermatological problems; 800 showed breaks and fractures; and another 325 represented deformities that had been corrected (Barreto n.d.). Fewer than 14 percent of the votive offerings were unrelated to illness and healing.

When Brazilians make a pilgrimage to the shrine of a saint, they are completing the central feature of what has become the model for the relationship between man and the supernatural copied in syncretic form by almost all of the country's other popular religions. They are performing acts of religious devotion that have been promised or bargained on the condition that they receive what was requested from the supernatural being. Since most requests are for healing, the very presence of a million or so pilgrims in Canindé every year, and the countless others who flock to the many pilgrimage sites throughout the country—not to speak of those in other parts of the world—indicates that the devotees believe they have recovered; they are no longer experiencing the symptoms that moved them to make their vows in the first place. In their eyes, they have been healed. Having obtained what they asked for, they now are delivering the veneration they promised as their part of the bargain with the supernatural.

CHAPTER 10

HEALING BY THE SPIRITS IN THE AFRICAN-DERIVED TRADITIONS

In the early sixteenth century, starting shortly after the official discovery and initial settlement of the lands of the Southern Cross that were to become Brazil, the Portuguese, following a model for colonization that had its origins in the eastern Mediterranean and was worked out in the islands of the Atlantic Ocean (see Greenfield 1979b, 1977a), brought slaves from West Africa to the Americas. The slaves provided the labor needed for the cultivation and processing of sugarcane, which was sold at great profit to consumers back in Europe. To adapt in the hostile new situation of bondage and servitude, those slaves who survived the perilous journey across the Atlantic Ocean undoubtedly turned for understanding and guidance to the beliefs of their home cultures. These worldviews were comprised of rich and varied cosmologies containing a variety of supernatural beings that were attributed causal efficacy in the affairs of this world.

The Portuguese expansion and the relationship of Portugal's citizens to other peoples—those they encountered in the trade of commodities overseas and those containeded in their far-flung colonization projects—were shaped by what today might be considered the extreme Christian principles that were common in most of Europe at the time. Slavery itself was justified in this system of religious beliefs because the eternal souls of "heathens" who resisted accepting Christ were being saved, even though the means employed and the human consequences might be considered deplorable.

Based on the Portuguese state's founding myth, the Crown and its religious missionaries instilled in colonists that they were bringing God's kingdom to what heretofore had been the domain of the devil. The king stood at the apex of the imperial system, with the administrative officers of the state, the clergy, and the plantation owners maintaining order and loyalty primarily by means of the largess they distributed. This patrimonial system of patronage, which satisfied at least the minimal needs of all sectors of the population, reinforced the belief in "hierarchy, order and paternalistic authority as socially inviolate and divinely preordained" (Pessar 2004:17).

Driven by this religiously oriented set of beliefs, slave owners in Brazil exposed their human chattels to, and usually forced them to accept, Christianity, which they did, albeit superficially in most cases. Often, as we have come to understand in retrospect, they hid the continuing worship of, and belief in, African deities—although not always the practices, which plantation overseers forced them to give up—behind the facade of the veneration of saints that was a basic aspect of the Christianity taught them and practiced by their masters. One common feature important for our purposes in these differing and sporadic instances of religious syncretism was the introduction into Brazilian religious practice, and its continuation across the many generations both before and after emancipation, of the African practice of spirit possession.

Europeans related to the supernatural through words in the form of prayer. In West Africa, by contrast, the gods, on being invoked by their devotees, came down from wherever they were assumed to be and incorporated in the bodies of the faithful. They took possession of special individuals trained to receive them and consequently were able to be, and interact with, the living.

The millions of slaves brought to Brazil over four centuries of trade came from a broad swath of western Africa, stretching from what today is Senegal in the north, south to the lands around the

Gulf of Guinea, and as far down as the former Portuguese colony of Angola. Hence a great number of the varied and diverse cultural and religious traditions of the peoples of western Africa became part of the local African-derived, syncretized religious traditions found throughout Brazil.

The descriptive details of the history of the interplay between Christianity and the multiple African traditions retained by the slaves have been mostly lost. What survived, by the time Catholicism ceased to be the official state faith of Brazil and religious diversity became legal after the advent of the republic in 1889, came to be known by many names in different parts of the country, each practice shaped by the specific cultural background of the African *nação* (nation) from which the forbearers of the local population had come.

These religions vary, in both their doctrines and their rituals. Each initiatic lineage is independent and not responsible to any superior body for the maintenance of conformity to a set of common traditions (Wafer 1991:4).

Three major forms of Candomblé are generally recognized. These are the Gêgê-Nagô tradition, the Angolan-Congo, and the Candomblés de Caboclo. Followers of the first claim it to be based on Yoruban and Fon languages and ethnic traditions; believers of the second derive their practices from Bantu origins; the third is an eclectic category that refers more to the mixture of deities worshipped than to the part of Africa from which the rituals derive. By the latter years of the twentieth century, for reasons partly touched on below, the Gêgê-Nagô tradition of the Yoruba and Fon peoples from what are now Nigeria and Benin, as practiced in the northeastern region of Brazil, specifically in the states of Bahia and Pernambuco, had surpassed the others in popular recognition and number of adherents.

The Gêgê-Nagô Candomblés were established in the late eighteenth/early nineteenth century in Salvador, presently the capital of the state of Bahia. Large numbers of slaves had been amassed there, having been brought by their owners from the interior plantations to be hired out in the commercial and service sectors when earnings from sugar, the primary commercial crop of the region, declined due to competition from more efficient producers elsewhere. The slaves, many of whom were first-generation arrivals, came primarily from the coastal areas of West Africa known as the Bight of Benin[22] (today the seacoasts of Ghana, Togo, Benin, and Nigeria), where they had shared similar cultures and linguistic forms. Nagô (as Yoruba was known in Brazil) was the primary language spoken by these slaves. It also served as the lingua franca in this part of the country (Verger 1976, 1964). When not actually working, the slaves would congregate in places provided by their owners where they were subjected to (considerably) less supervision than on the plantations. It was here that they are believed to have been able to practice rituals that were part of the belief system still remembered by many from the time before their capture (Harding 2000).

Two free women, both of Nagô, or Yoruba, origin, are reported to have founded the first terreiro, or separate space for the practice of what was to be called Candomblé. Soon other places—known as houses—were opened. Small numbers of slaves, and then freedmen from Africa or of African descent, although marginal and insignificant with respect to the larger society, were able to participate in activities that through the efforts of scholars and intellectuals—as much as their own leaders—came to be viewed as "pure" or "authentic African" religious practices. Under comparable conditions, additional places, not all based on Yoruba tradition, soon appeared in other parts of the country. Although the police harassed the practitioners of these pejoratively called "cults," and leaders of the formal church put pressure on the civil authorities to have them closed, the terreiros resisted and survived. All told, the number of people participating in the Candomblés and other African-derived, or Afro-Brazilian, religions (known variously by names such as Xangô, Macumba, Batuque, and Tambor de Minas) was small. These religions of the feast, as they have been called, are characterized today by animal sacrifice, divination, trance, and incorporation and possession by gods from Africa, who dance to the rhythm of drums and interact with their devotees, guide their lives, and enter into exchanges with them (Motta 2001, 1982).

From their beginnings through the middle of the twentieth century, the African-derived religions of Brazil, in all of their varying forms, were practiced by small numbers of mostly descendants of Africans who were marginal to the larger society. The catalyst for their becoming widely practiced and being projected onto the national scene, according to Prandi (1991), was the counterculture movement of the 1960s, when Brazil was undergoing the turmoil of rapid urbanization and industrialization and its government was in the hands of the military, which had seized power in a coup in 1964. Like their contemporaries throughout the world, but with special focus on, and reaction to, the oppression being inflicted under the military dictatorship, intellectuals and young, mostly educated members of the middle classes rebelled, not so much physically but by seeking solutions to the problems of their world in the mystical cultures and practices of others. Some turned to the traditions of India, China, and the Middle East, but still more looked to the "Negro" cultures of their own northeast that were beginning to be known through the increasing popularity of Umbanda (see chapter 11).

A fast-growing media industry disseminated information about the range of African-derived religions, whose "consumers" were of many diverse ethnicities. In addition to Afro-Brazilians of all degrees of racial mixture, descendants of the early Iberians and later immigrants from Italy, Germany, Poland, and elsewhere on the European continent, plus those from the Middle East and Asia,[23] learned about African religion through songs and stories, on records, radio, and television. Since most media coverage, and that by scholars, especially anthropologists, focused on the terreiros of Salvador and other areas of Nagô influence as its source, African-derived religion in Brazil came to be heavily Yoruba-centric (Motta 1998; Dantas 1988).

New terreiros, which soon would provide places for the reinterpreted and Brazilianized "beliefs from Africa," appeared. Many Umbanda centers reincorporated "more African" elements made known in the media and attracted a general public that was to seek in them solutions to their formidable problems. Enterprising heads of some São Paulo and Rio de Janeiro terreiros went to Salvador to be formally initiated by the (black and mostly female) heads of the older and more prestigious houses, thereby making their terreiros part of a newly created network of "authentic" Afro-Brazilian centers through a form of ritualized fictive kinship, since each became a son or daughter (*filho* or *filha*) of a Bahian *pai-* or *mãe-de-santo* (father or mother in sainthood). Meanwhile, the leaders of these "authentic" centers, with the help of sympathetic intellectuals, attempted to make Candomblé an "official" religion, with a status on par with the

Catholic Church, by denying the syncretic aspects of its history (see Wafer 1991:56; Dantas 1982).

The number of terreiros throughout the country increased dramatically and served Brazilians of African descent in addition to members of the population from all classes, races, and ethnicities. As in São Paulo and Rio de Janeiro, descendants of European immigrants, as far south as the state of Rio Grande do Sul, which borders Argentina and Uruguay, started participating in the growing number of Afro-Brazilian religious centers. Oro (1988) reports, from a survey of terreiros in greater Porto Alegre, that hundreds of people of Italian and German descent were already participating in Afro-Brazilian religions and comprised 4.1 percent of the heads of the more than 11,000 registered centers. The leader of one of the federations of Afro-Brazilian religions was the son of an Italian immigrant (see also Greenfield 1994). By the end of the twentieth century, the majority of the heads of what Oro (1999) calls the "popular terreiros" were white.[24]

At the center she studied in Belém, the motivation for the initial participation of newcomers, writes Cohen (2007:53), citing its pai-de-santo, is "a deliberate response to troublesome, negative, and detrimental life circumstances":

> The wide variety of … issues that bring clients to the terreiro can be condensed to three main themes: love, money and health. ….
> No one arrives at his consultation desk in search of a new philosophy, or having been informed or inspired by Afro-Brazilian theology. Essentially, first time clients suspect that there is something unnatural about their sudden or unabated, unhappy state of affairs, or at least suppose that their best hope of bettering their situation, having "tried everything else," is by methods that invoke supernatural powers. …The rituals that a client may have to perform are relatively simple, means-to-end procedures. (Cohen 2007:53–54).

In an example, representative of the broader process of new adepts (in this case not of African descent) being recruited in exchange for healing, an Italian emigrant from a small interior town in Calabria told me the following story. She had married a local boy at the age of eighteen. Both had traveled to Brazil in 1925 at the invitation of the boy's father, who already was there.

Several years later, when Maria was pregnant with her second child, her husband (whose father had died) abandoned her. When the baby, Luiz, was two months old, he took seriously ill. The doctors were unable to help. The desperate mother, following the advice of a friend, took the boy to a mãe-de-santo—described as *bem pretinha* (very dark skinned) and a *filha de Xangô* (a daugher of the Yoruba deity Xangô).

Luiz recovered in three days, after which his mother did something not unusual for a Catholic woman who believed that she had been the recipient of a miracle: she promised her son to God. In this case, however, she promised the boy not to the Roman Catholic Church but to the gods of Africa who had helped her son in response to her request.

Maria did not tell the boy the story but did take him to Batuque and Umbanda centers, where he participated in ritual activities. Until he was fourteen, Luiz claimed he wanted to be a priest. At fifteen he decided instead to take training at an Umbanda center. Two years later, changing his mind once more, he went to live with the woman whose deity had saved his life. By the time he was eighteen, he had been initiated by her in Batuque. Only then did Maria tell him about his childhood illness and the promise she had made on his recovery. Luiz later opened his own center, where his mother is an initiate. Both identify not as Brazilians but as Italians living in Brazil devoted to the "gods" of Africa. Maria says that they brought her to Brazil so she could learn about them and engage in their rituals (Greenfield 1994).

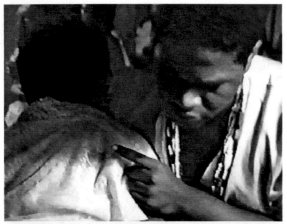

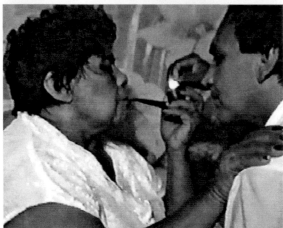

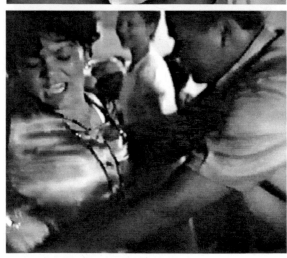

(Top) Mediums incorporated by deities greeting each other. (Middle) Mãe-de-santo during consultation with a client. (Bottom) Mediums in trance incorporating specific deities.

CHAPTER 11

HEALING IN UMBANDA

Umbanda, a mixture of the various religious strains already discussed, is said to have first appeared in the opening decade of the twentieth century. According to Brown ([1986] 1994:37ff), Umbanda was part of an intentional effort by a unique and farsighted group of middle-class Brazilians, who happened to be Kardecists, seeking to create a distinct, unifying belief system that would bring together the peoples of different national, racial, cultural, and religious backgrounds. These were the citizens of the new Brazilian nation.

The defining moment, according to what may be considered Umbanda's origin myth, took place at a Kardecist-Spiritist center in Niteroi, a city across Guanabara Bay from Rio de Janeiro. There, a tall, blond, white-skinned young man named Zélio de Morais reportedly received the spirit of a mixed Indian and Afro-Brazilian, the Caboclo das Sete Encruzilhadas (the Spirit of the Seven Crossroads), who instructed him to found a new religion (St. Clair 1971:136). The next day, Morais received a preto velho (the spirit of an African slave), who repeated the instructions (Trinidade 1989:ch. 3). Kardecists until then did not acknowledge that the enlightenment they sought in their encounters with beings from the other world could be obtained from spirits who had not been Europeans in their previous lifetimes.

The first decade of the twentieth century was a period of intellectual ferment in Brazil. An educated elite was trying to provide the new republican regime with symbols and an image of national unity and identity. Less than two decades earlier, in 1889, the emperor, who had reigned over Brazil since it had gained its independence from Portugal under his father in 1822, had been replaced—in a bloodless revolution—by a republican government based on a constitution modeled on that of the United States. The intellectuals used this political-administrative transformation to proclaim the arrival of a democratic Brazil, based not on its actual social and political life but on their minimal understanding of the culture and society of their North American neighbor. Brazil was a democracy in name only at the turn of the twentieth century. Though competitive elections held under its post military constitution and recent governments have made the nation considerably more democratic, Brazil was then, and still is, in many deep-seated respects, a nation that is patrimonial, patriarchal, and ordered hierarchically. Social relations continue to be based on patron–client exchanges and relationships derived from the symbolic dynamic in the promessas and payments of pilgrims analyzed above (see also Greenfield and Cavalcante 2006; Roniger 1990, 1987; Greenfield 1979a, 1977b, 1972; Hutchinson 1966).

Although slavery had been abolished in 1888, only a year before the new political system was put in place, for the quarter of a century prior, emigrants had been arriving in São Paulo and the states to its south in increasing numbers in a deliberate effort by the imperial government to transform the physical makeup of the national population from peoples of color, primarily of African descent, to Europeans. Racist thinking, very much in vogue at the time, presented Brazil's new image makers with a dilemma that gave rise to another bit of wishful thinking. Nonwhites were considered by the educated elites to be inferior and incapable of developing an advanced or modern nation, which Brazil aspired to be. To counter this notion, the intellectuals invented another myth: that their country was a racial democracy that had been formed by the mixing, both physical and cultural—since biology and culture were fused in racist beliefs—of its founding populations of Europeans, Africans, and Indians (Maggie 1996). Furthermore, they maintained, the nonwhite population would mix with the European immigrants to "whiten"—again both physically and culturally—the future citizens of the nation (Maio and Santos 1996:part I).

Morais, who had been raised a Catholic (like so many other

Brazilians at that time and now), had frequented Macumba, as the Afro-Brazilian syncretism prevalent in Rio de Janeiro was known. The Caboclo das Sete Encruzilhadas is said to have told Morais that none of the other religions being practiced in the nation was right, and it "proceeded to dictate a brand-new set of rules, regulations, rituals, chants, drumbeats, herbal cures, curses, dance steps, etc." (St. Clair 1971:136). The product of the "revelation" was a distinctive mixed or syncretized religion that would, it was claimed by its followers, satisfy the needs of the new national society being created.

To clarify the role of healing in the religion and the place of spirit possession within it, I turn to some case materials that I collected in Rio de Janeiro during several sojourns there in the 1980s and 1990s. These descriptions are injected to provide an example of the growth and popularity of Umbanda.

At 5:30 p.m., on a Thursday evening at Cabelos Unisex Joanna, a hair-styling salon in the still-fashionable Copacabana section of Rio de Janeiro, Celestina de Araujo Santos, a pretty young woman of twenty-two, with dark eyes, long black hair, and a captivating smile, was cleaning up the work area where she had spent the day shampooing, cutting, and setting the hair of middle-class clients. She was hurriedly preparing to leave before 6:00 p.m. without upsetting Dona Joanna, the owner of the shop, who liked to sit around and gossip with her employees over coffee after the doors were closed to customers. Celestina had an important appointment later in the evening that she did not want to discuss with Dona Joanna or her coworkers. She had to be at the Casa de Vovô Maria, an Umbanda center way out in the Baxada Fluminese, the lowlands between the coastal mountains to the northwest of the city, before 7:30 p.m. The bus ride at the height of the evening rush would take well over an hour, and there would be a long line to wait on at the bus stop.

Celestina had been attending sessions at the Umbanda center for exactly six months, ever since her cousin had brought her there. Although she had successfully completed the training program that qualified her for her job with Dona Joanna only a month earlier, and she loved the work and was doing quite well at it, she was in the process of breaking up with her boyfriend. She had also developed back pains that made it difficult for her to stand all day and be pleasant and perky with the customers.

She had gone to the public health clinic near the *favela* (squatter settlement), where she lived with her parents, to seek relief from the back pains. There, after a several-hour wait and a brief, superficial examination, a doctor gave her a prescription for medications, which she dutifully filled at the pharmacy near work, in spite of the very high cost. But after taking the pills as prescribed for the requisite period, she felt no better. In too much pain to go to work one day, she told her cousin about her problems, including the fights with her boyfriend. Neda suggested that Celestina accompany her to the Casa de Vovô Maria on the next night, which was a Thursday, when they had sessions open to the public, to seek the advice and help of Mãe Edna and her spirits. Neda told her cousin how she had been helped with an even more serious problem by the mãe-de-santo and her *pomba gira* (spirit guide), as had several of her friends.

Raised as a Roman Catholic, Celestina resisted at first but then acquiesced, perhaps out of desperation, and accompanied her cousin on Thursday. Tonight she would be going again, this time to commit to a training program through which she would learn to serve the spirits so that someday she would be able to help others as she herself had been helped. That's why she had to be there by 7:30 p.m., when the ritual singing and dancing known as the *gira* began. Mãe Edna did not like her *filhos-* and *filhas-de-santo (*saint sons and daughters) to arrive late. And since Celestina was to become a daughter of the house, she wished to arrive before the ritual began, in time to change from the short skirt and colorful blouse she wore for work into the clean white outfit, with its numerous starched petticoats, that was packed in the worn old valise she had borrowed from her mother. The bag was tucked away in the corner near the area that she was busily trying to make spotless to satisfy Dona Joanna. It also contained a special outfit that Celestina had purchased only the day before, after saving up the money by skimping on meals and other basics for several weeks. It was the costume of Iemanjá, the goddess that Mãe Edna had told her was one of the "owners of her head," as an individual's personal spirit guide is called in Umbanda. Celestina was planning to wear the costume that night, changing into it just before the *ponto,* the ritual song invoking the spirit, was sung. She hoped that Iemanjá would honor her by incorporating into and possessing her body if she entered into trance for the first of what she hoped would be many times.

The young beautician arrived in time, just before 7:30 p.m., as the large hall in the deceptive-looking building that stretched back off the street was being cleansed with incense and rose petals. Celestina changed her clothes.

A sense of heightened expectation filled the air as a short, dark-skinned, heavyset woman in her late fifties, dressed in a white blouse and white fluffed skirt supported by a heavily starched cotton pettiskirt (or underskirt), started to sing, dance, and clap her hands. As her body gyrated rhythmically, with her barefooted steps moving her sideways in a counterclockwise direction, some fifteen white-clad men and women joined her. Three men at the side of the room, also clothed in white, soon were accompanying them on drums. Almost a hundred people, seated on bare benches behind a railing that divided the room, swayed and moved to the beat of the rhythm. They were of all ages and racial combinations. Although most were mature women, more than one-third were children and adult men.

The words of the song that opened the ritual were an invocation, first to God and then to "Our Lady." Prayers to a number of spirit beings, ranging from the African orixás to Kardecist spirits of light to pretos velhoss, caboclos, and exus followed. A Catholic blessing was recited, and a passage from *The Spirit's Book* by Allan Kardec was read.

After a brief pause, the lead woman resumed her rhythmic beat. This time it was a ponto invoking the African god Xangô (believed by some to be the Roman Catholic St. Jerome), imploring him to come down and be with his devotees. Within minutes, one of the dancers, Marco Antônio dos Santos, began to spin rapidly. His body shook violently in a series of spasms. The dark-skinned woman and a tall, thin, mulatto man, who had been standing behind the circle of dancers, quickly came to his side. After removing the man's wristwatch and other jewelry, they guided his movements. His gyrating body pulsated, taking him deeper into trance. A sudden, almost uncontrollable jerk backward was acknowledged by the others as the sign that the deity had entered his body. Xangô/St. Jerome, now manifest in his "horse" and dancing wildly in the midst of his devotees, was greeted with his own special cry, *"Caô cabecile."*

Like Marco Antônio, other mediums in the gira were soon spinning and shaking, as one by one each went into trance and received (incorporated) a series of deities. Every manifestation was greeted with the cry of "Caô cabecile," followed by the touching of shoulders, first the right to the right of the facing person, then the left shoulder to the left. Under the supervising eye of the ritual leader and the tall man who was her second in command (a pai-de-santo), the bare-footed dancers began "giving themselves up" to Xangô/St. Jerome. In turn, they greeted first the ritual leader, then her assistant, then the others who had entered into trance, and finally everyone else in the circle of dancers.

The ritualized singing, dancing, drumming, and greetings continued for approximately thirty minutes. Then one after another of the pos-sessed mediums jerked backward violently, indicating that Xangô/St. Jerome had left them to return to the spirit world. Once out of trance, some mediums walked slowly to the side of the room. Others contin-ued to follow the beat until the drumming and chanting stopped.

Following a brief pause, the mãe-de-santo began to sing anoth-er ponto, invoking a second deity. The drummers took up the new rhythm immediately. Many of those seated on the benches joined in the song as those in front of the railing formed the characteris-tic circle. In the next few hours, Ogun/St. George, Iemanjá/Our Lady of Glory, Obaluaé /St. Lazarus, Iansã/St. Barbara, and other orixás/saints descended and incorporated in reply to the requests in the words of their pontos.

According to Umbanda theology, the orixás/saints serve as pro-tector spirits for their devotees, who are referred to as their filhos (children). Each human being, in a carryover of Yoruba cosmology mixed with popular Catholicism, is believed to be assigned at birth to one of the orixás/saints. The identity of one's protector can be dis-covered by means of divination, the reading of cowry shells that are tossed in a practice also of African provenience.

At about 10:00 p.m., there was a break in the service. The saint mother and the other mediums had quietly left the large room and were no longer to be seen. Those seated on the benches stirred but did not attempt to leave. A heightening sense of tension engulfed the hall as the minutes passed. Then, reminiscent of what we have seen at Kardecist rituals, ushers approached those waiting behind the railing and asked them to look at the number on the *ficha* (token) they had been given when they first entered the center that evening. Each person had a colored number that corresponded to the name of the spirit with whom he or she wished to consult. The deities, unique to the expanded pantheon of Umbanda, were all spirits of the dead drawn from stereotyped social categories prominent in popular

Brazilian history. They included: 1) pretos velhoss, or spirits of wise, loyal old slaves; 2) caboclos, spirits of independent and still defiant Indians; 3) exus, a category including rogues, thieves, prostitutes, gypsies, and other colorful characters familiar to most members of the national society, especially the poor; and 4) crianças, spirits of children representing the racially and culturally mixed and unified Brazilians of the future hoped for by Umbanda's founders.

Marco Antônio, the young man to enter trance first that evening, had changed his clothes and was now wearing a pair of old, faded blue jeans and a threadbare striped shirt. He was seated in a tiny alcove in a second building much older than the one into which the orixás/saints had descended. On the floor before him were a number of small statues, a burning candle, and an empty water glass. As he prepared to go into trance and receive Pai Joaquim, his preto velho, he reflected on the day a few years previously when he had first come to the Casa de Vovô Maria. He had been physically ill. He had gone to the doctor and taken medical tests, but no diagnosis could be given for his complaints of excessive fatigue, nagging pains in his back and shoulders, lack of appetite, and general despondency. Adequate help could not be provided. Things were constantly going wrong at work. He had been fighting with his girlfriend, who had become involved with someone else, he believed. He felt that his life was at an impasse.

A colleague at the bank where he worked had first mentioned Mãe Edna and her Umbanda center. The man explained how medical doctors had been unable to cure his youngest child when she was ill. After several traumatic incidents, a neighbor suggested that Maria Padilha, the pomba gira that Mãe Edna received and after whom her center was named, might be able to aid the child. The father told Marco Antônio about the child's recovery after being treated at the Umbanda center. Not knowing what else to do, the young bank clerk went to a public session like the one Celestina had attended.

He remembered his skepticism when he first saw Mãe Edna and the filhos and filhas-de-santo sing and dance and go into trance. After all, he was an intelligent and educated person with a university degree. He should have known better than to participate in such *brucharia* (witchcraft), as his father had called it when his son told him of his decision to attend the session.

Nevertheless, he decided to consult with the pomba gira. After the last of the orixás/saints incorporated and then departed, he waited as assistants led others out of the room. Marco Antônio was tempted to run for home until finally a young woman approached him, calling out the number on the red ficha he held in his hand. He followed her to a small room, where others were waiting to ask advice from Maria Padilha. As he gradually moved forward on the line, he saw Mãe Edna, who was dressed in the attire of what to him seemed to be a nineteenth-century prostitute. She smoked a cigarette in a long black holder and gulped liquid from a champagne glass being refilled—for the fourth time since he had entered the room—by an attendant. When his turn finally came, she greeted him in a deep, sultry voice, in an accent he could scarcely understand, and asked what his problem was and how she might help him. Although he recognized her, since he had seen her just a few minutes before in the outer room, her looks and behavior were very different from what he had previously noted.

In a flirtatious, thickly accented tone, she promised to help rid him of his symptoms. She said he would have to return for a private session and bring with him live chickens, a goat, and other small animals. She enumerated a list for him. The *trabalho* (work) would cost what at the time amounted to several hundred dollars. It would take Marco Antônio more than a month to save that much money.

The young clerk tried to put the matter out of his mind, but Sr. Caitano, his colleague at the bank, would not let him. Furthermore, Sr. Caitano offered to help obtain the necessary items and to accompany Marco Antônio when he returned to the center. A few days prior to the scheduled date, the still ill and despondent young man had just about decided not to go, but when he grew even more fatigued and the pains increased, in spite of the medication the doctor prescribed, he changed his mind. Over the objections of his "very Catholic" father, he purchased the animals and went to have the work done for him by the pomba gira.

When he arrived at the religious center late on a Tuesday afternoon, Mãe Edna was already in trance. It was Maria Padilha who asked if he brought the offerings. She informed him that his paths were closed and that her efforts would help to open them, leading eventually to his recovery. She took the animals he had purchased and, with the help of several other adepts who were also in trance, sacrificed them ritually by slitting their throats with a special knife. Selected parts of the animals, along with some of the other items he had brought, were used to prepare what he was told were the favorite foods of specific orixás/saints and exus who would resolve his problems. The pomba gira also informed Marco Antônio that he had mediumship ability that he would have to develop if he wished to recover completely. This could be accomplished by taking a training program at any Umbanda center where it was offered. The implication, as he came to understand, was that to be cured, he would have to learn to receive the spirits of orixás/saints, pretos velhos, caboclos, exus, and crianças. He would be obliged to contribute his body and his being to Umbanda's program of training mediums to be available to the spirits so that they might interact with, heal, and otherwise help those in need. In brief, he would have to become an Umbandista and be possessed by Umbanda's spirits.

In the days following the trabalho, Marco Antônio's pains, to his and his skeptical father's great surprise, gradually subsided. He had more energy. His appetite returned. He slept at night for the first time in months and no longer felt depressed.

That had been three years earlier. Since then he had become one of a growing number of regulars at the center. Recently, he had completed his first *obrigação* (obligation), beginning the initiatory cycle that would lead to his eventually qualifying to direct his own Umbanda center. For now he remained a spiritual son of Mãe Edna. As her filho, he contributed to her enterprise by serving as a horse for the orixás/saints and by giving his body to Pai Joaquim, his preto velho, who helped others as he himself had been helped.

As he began to experience the sensations that signaled the arrival of Pai Joaquim, Marco Antônio knew that he would not remember what would transpire while he was possessed by the supernatural being. He could not recall the period earlier in the evening when he had incorporated Xangô, Ogun, Iemanjá and the other orixás/saints. Mãe Edna or Pai André, the tall thin man who was her second in command, would tell him what had happened and in doing so make suggestions that would enable him to improve himself as a medium. But in private sessions when he performed the charity of healing, when they were not watching since they were possessed by their own entities that were attending clients, he was alone. He wondered what was being said and done that made so many of those who consulted with him return and become part of the religious community.

Celestina de Araujo Santos remembered that on her first visit to the Casa de Vovô Maria, as she approached the alcove to consult with

Pai Joaquim, she had been startled by what she witnessed. In the dim light, she saw a slender, athletic young man appear to become instantaneously old and frail. As she walked down the corridor toward him, the medium's body seemed to shrink and age before her eyes. Although still tall for a Brazilian, he looked several inches shorter than he had been when she had entered the room. His limber frame had become bent and curved. He dragged his left foot, which now appeared to be almost useless, as he turned to sit on a stool placed behind the statues and the burning candle. When he rose later, he used a cane that was resting under the stool. To Celestina, the man with whom she was about to consult, who had been young and vigorous when she entered the hall, now seemed shriveled up and aged.

An assistant struck a match as the figure haltingly picked up a pipe and raised it toward his mouth. The aid filled the glass on the floor with *cachaça,* raw rum that Marco Antônio was known to despise. The bank clerk neither drank nor smoked, but when he worked at the center as a medium for Pai Joaquim, his body consumed as much as two liters of cachaça and an eight-ounce pouch of tobacco. He did not remember the smoking and drinking when he came out of trance; he also felt no ill effects from the tobacco and alcohol.

After taking a few puffs on the pipe and downing half of the glass of alcohol, the figure had asked the anxious Celestina how he could help her. His heavily accented words were spoken slowly and deliberately. Many of the expressions he used were not part of present-day Portuguese as it is currently spoken in Brazil. The assistant translated for the client. Relieved and grateful for the help, Celestina told the embodied medium about her back pains and problems with her boyfriend.

The preto velho invited the client to return to the center two weeks hence. Then, private work that would resolve her problem would be performed. At that time the young beautician, like Marco Antônio and countless others before and after her, was told that she had mediumship ability that she would have to develop to be fully healed. Like so many who had been helped by an Umbanda deity, Celestina did the work recommended by Pai Joaquim. In addition she embarked on the training program that culminated in her presence this evening to begin a career as an Umbanda adept, receiving its deities and participating in rituals as a medium for an assortment of syncretized spirit beings that cure and otherwise help the sick in exchange for their adherence to, and participation in, the new religion.

CHAPTER 12

EVANGELICALS AND HEALING BY THE HOLY GHOST

The final religious group competing for followers in the Brazilian religious marketplace to be discussed came to South America from the United States. Protestants tried to break the nation's Catholic monopoly twice in the early years—initially, in 1557, when French Huguenots settled on the shores of Guanabara Bay, and again in 1624, when Dutch Calvinists conquered Olinda, Recife, and Bahía in the Northeast. On both occasions, they were repulsed and driven out. Their houses of worship were confiscated and made the property of the Catholic Church.

In return for aiding the flight of the Portuguese royal family from Lisbon to Rio de Janeiro to escape Napoleon's advancing armies at the beginning of the nineteenth century, the British secured a treaty permitting the Anglican Church to enter Brazilian territory. Two years after independence, Emperor Dom Pedro I arranged for German Lutherans to settle in the contested southern borderlands with Spain, raise crops for themselves, and defend the territory for the new Brazilian state. Pastors, brought from Europe, were allowed to minister to the new Protestant subjects. With the door now open, in 1835 the Board of Foreign Missions of the Methodist Episcopal Church in the United States sent its first missionary to Rio de Janeiro.[25]

Beginning in 1850, the Southern Baptist Convention realized the potential for soul saving in this first independent and largest South American nation. After the reverends Daniel P. Kidder and James C. Fletcher visited and published a book in English about Brazil (1857), some American southerners—plantation- and slave-owning Protestants who feared the loss of their way of life with a victory by the North in the Civil War—relocated to Brazil. Some went to the Amazon, but most settled in the areas around the then small city of São Paulo. These Presbyterians, Baptists, and Methodists organized churches and petitioned their homeland for pastors.

Pentecostalism, the fastest growing and most prominent form of Protestantism in the competition for modern converts, arrived in Brazil differently. Unaffiliated missionaries from the United States came to spread the then new form of Protestantism, initially to the poor and later to immigrants, locating first in the hinterlands and eventually in the urban, industrializing centers of the country.

Modern Pentecostalism is considered by some to be the product of the message first preached by William Joseph Seymour, while other church people believe its beginnings to be in the nineteenth-century Holiness movement,[26] In April 1906, Seymour, an itinerant African American preacher, was invited to officiate at a church in Los Angeles (Anderson 2004:ch. 2; Chestnut 1997:25).[27] He used the occasion to expound a doctrine based in part on the beliefs of Holiness spirituality, to which he had converted in 1900. Based on an event in the book of Acts, "in which the Holy Spirit descended on the apostles in tongues of fire, causing them to preach in languages previously unknown to them," the preacher claimed that similarly all those to accept the faith would be possessed by the Holy Spirit during spiritual baptism (Chestnut 1997:176). Moreover, "as the prophet Joel had foretold, the gifts of healing, ecstasy, tongues, and prophecy, enjoyed by the Primitive Church would be restored to the people of God immediately before the Last Days" (Armstrong 2000:179). Seymour taught that Christians should read and accept as literally true what was written in the Bible (Westmeier 1999:20). He preached that the end of days was imminent and that each person to receive the Holy Spirit was obligated to spread the message.

The first congregants did not respond positively to Seymour or his message. When he was locked out of the Los Angeles church, he began home prayer meetings, where he continued to preach the gifts of the Holy Spirit and the imminence of the apocalypse (Chestnut 1997:25). News of the San Francisco earthquake led many who had rejected Seymour's message to reconsider, igniting what Chestnut refers to as "the Pentecostal conflagration that rages across the globe almost a century later" (1997:26).

Within five years of the event in California, Pentecostalism had spread across the United States and beyond. In 1911 two Swedish immigrants, Gunnar Vingren and Daniel Berg, who had settled in South Bend, Indiana, departed to fulfill the prophecy they had received.[28] Landing in the tropical port city of Belém at the mouth of Brazil's Amazon River on a third-class steamer, they worked in harmony with a Baptist pastor until they gained their first convert. When their disciple spoke in tongues, after being baptized in the Holy Spirit following an act of faith healing, a chain of events began. That chain "culminated in a church schism and the birth of what was to become the Western Hemisphere's largest Pentecostal denomination, the Assembléia de Deus (the Assembly of God)" (Chestnut 1997:27).

A year before Vingren and Berg came to Belém, Luis Francescon, an Italian who had immigrated to the United States and converted to Pentecostalism in Chicago, landed in São Paulo to fulfill his own prophecy. Invited to preach (in Italian) at a Presbyterian church in a neighborhood of working-class Italian immigrants, he too was forced to leave when his converts began to speak in tongues. Francescon established his own church called the Congregação Christã (Christian Congregation).

From these inauspicious beginnings, Pentecostalism spread slowly throughout Brazil. By 1936, twenty-five years after the founding of the first church, Protestant denominations, established and administered by foreign missionaries, with close ties to their churches at home, had made little headway and gained relatively few converts. Hence they remained small, marginal groups.

After 1936 Pentecostalism grew more quickly, led by the Asembléia de Deus (AD) and the Congregação Christã (CC).[29] According to Donald Curry (n.d.), two things were necessary for this growth to happen: Brazilian nationals had to take over the churches and then had to sever their ties of dependency with home operations.[30] Native Brazilian missionaries moved to the hinterlands and blazed a trail of backwoods Protestantism that extended from the mule-trading center of Sorocaba, west of São Paulo, down the length of the coffee zone in the valley of the Paraíba River. There the missionaries copied the pattern of settlement and growth employed by those (read Roman Catholics) who had preceded them in successfully set- tling the Brazilian interior (see Curry n.d.:92; Ferreira 1959:vol. 1, 30–34). While "frontier revivalism" flourished in the United States, Brazilian Pentecostals and other Protestants diverged from the practices of their North American founders by copying and replicating the "'Mediterranean' rules of city-founding" that had operated in Brazil since its first settlement (Curry n.d.:93). As Curry (n.d.:95ff) describes the pattern, an itinerant preacher moved into an uncultivated and uninhabited region opened for a new cash crop and brought followers to settle and cultivate land he had obtained in the name of the church. Using contacts with bankers in the regional center where the church had its seat (*sede*), he obtained loans for his parishioners. Like his secular counterparts, the preacher brokered the sale of the crops harvested by his fellow *crentes*, as Protestants are called, and served as a commercial middleman, with profits accruing to the church. Once the economic enterprise (the *feitoria*, or "factory") produced income, the preacher negotiated the votes of his flock in exchange for the support of a local political power broker. The *prefeito* (mayor) of the municipality, president of the *camara de vereadores* (municipal council), or a deputy in the state legislature (if the preacher was lucky) established a place for him and his group in the local political arena. The preacher gained official designation as pastor in charge of the church built by his followers in the sede (in this case the urban center of the municipality) dominated by the political leader the group supported. "The basic plan of a mayor-and-council, upon which the *município* system was founded," Curry continues, "is replicated among the Protestants in the pastor-and-council" (n.d.:99). The Brazilian mayor was a strong figure with "almost dictatorial power after election. The Protestant pastor had ... the same kind of authority." He presided as the chief of a "corporation" that held considerable amounts of property, and he used his subordinates in the furtherance of his own career (see Chestnut 1997; Mariz 1994 for examples). Moreover, like the mayor of a municipality, he was expected to mediate between the local city administration and the state for the redistribution of emoluments and rewards, patronage for his church and the members of his flock.

Evidence of the success of this adoption of the Brazilian (Catholic) organizational pattern is found in the number of converts preachers were able to attract. From 1932 to the mid-1950s, Chestnut tells us, "twenty-nine times more believers claimed Pentecostal affiliation" (1997:31, citing Endruveit).

In the 1950s, another wave of Pentecostal missionary activity arrived from the United States to establish a third important church. In 1922 Canadian evangelist Aimee Semple McPherson had founded the International Church of the Foursquare Gospel, where she integrated Hollywood showmanship into evangelistic campaigns. McPherson pioneered the use of radio and by 1924 had her own station. She toured the country, filling tents and auditoriums, deemphasizing the ascetic codes of conduct of traditional Pentecostalism, and instead offering "the promise of healing for the physically ill and those afflicted by the economic demons of the Great Depression" (Chestnut 1997:35).

In 1953 Harold Williams, a film actor turned missionary and a disciple of McPherson, brought the Foursquare Gospel to Brazil. With Raymond Boatright, another American entertainer turned preacher, belting out gospel hymns to rock rhythms on the electric guitar, he launched a National Evangelization Crusade in São Paulo using the quintessentially North American tent revival. Opposition by local Brazilian Pentecostal leaders brought the crusade to a premature end, but Williams founded the Crusade Church (Igreja Cruzada), which was reorganized the following year as the Igreja do Evangelho Quadrangular (IEQ) under primarily Brazilian leadership. While making few converts until the 1970s, the IEQ provided a modern motif to the Pentecostal message in Brazil. Collective faith healing sessions, which formed the core of Seymour's and McPherson's ministries in the United States and the heart of Williams and Boatright's crusade, were the primary recruiting technique of the IEQ (Chestnut 1997:35).

Manoel de Mello, a charismatic lay preacher and popular healer from the state of Pernambuco in the northeast, left the AD to join the National Evangelization Crusade and rose quickly to national prominence by performing miraculous healings. Mello's great popularity quickly transcended the crusade, leading him to found his own church, Brasil para Cristo (BPC), in 1955 (Read 1965:144–45). On the model of the crusade, he and the BPC took the message to rented stadiums, theaters, auditoriums, and gymnasiums (Freston 1993:87). Mello started a radio program on which he sang hymns set to the rhythms of the northeast. This proved to be very popular with the many migrants from that region who relocated to São Paulo in the following years.

Mello adapted the earlier church practice of participating in politics to the large urban setting. In exchange for a generous piece of city property on which to build a temple, he brokered the votes of his many followers in the BPC to Ademar de Barros in his campaign for presidency of the republic. Mello announced a "gift" from the federal deputy to the church's estimated five million members on his radio program and organized all-night prayer vigils at which "worshippers implored the Holy Ghost to aid in Barros's election" (Chestnut 1997:37).

Though Barros lost the election, he remained a federal deputy. So as not to further offend the Catholic Church, and without any warning, the shrewd politician had Mello's newly constructed temple razed (Read 1965:151). Undaunted, the astute minister marshaled his flock to elect his assistant, Levy Tavares, federal deputy and another BPC pastor state deputy.

In a classic pattern of Pentecostal schismatic growth, David Miranda left the BPC in 1962 to start the Igreja Pentecostal Deus É Amor (God Is Love Pentecostal Church; DEA). Unlike the other rather free and loose new Pentecostal groups in São Paulo, he reimposed strict controls over dress, personal conduct, and relations between the sexes. Miranda emphasized faith healing, elevating his church to an "agency of divine healing" (Mendonça and Velsques Filho 1990).

Shunning the new medium of television, Miranda depended on the radio. At the end of the 1970s, his daily *Voz da Libertação* (Voice of Liberation) radio program was broadcast on more than five hundred stations, including at least five that he owned personally (Landim 1989:62).

Borrowing from popular Catholicism and the range of African-derived religions, "God is Love recovered the thaumaturgy eliminated centuries ago by the Protestant Reformers" (Chestnut 1997:38). Exorcism, used to expel demons from their human hosts and invoke the "evil African spirits" of so many of the other competitors in the marketplace, became a main activity of DEA. Visual imagery replaced the extreme austerity of classic Pentecostal houses of worship.

In 1977 Edir Macedo, a lottery employee from Rio de Janeiro, founded the *igreja* Universal do Reino de Deus (the Universal Church of the Kingdom of God; IURD), which was to become the quintessential example of a Brazilian Pentecostal church and arguably one of Brazil's more unusual multinational corporations. An eclectic range of religious experiences, not unusual for a Brazilian living in a metropolitan center during the 1970s and 1980s, made Macedo keenly aware of the importance of the helping activities of the Kardecist spirits, African orixás, Umbanda exus, pretos-velho, and caboclos in the successes of his competitors. The growth of popular Catholicism, with its emphasis on the saints assisting those who made promessas to them, and the increase in numbers of followers of Candomblé, Umbanda, and Kardecism who had been cured by their supernatural entities clearly demonstrated this point. So it is not surprising, since the most common and frequently provided form of assistance offered by all the churches was healing, that Macedo placed the miraculous healing of the Holy Ghost as the keystone of his ministry (see also Greenfield 2002). Like the other churches, the new ministry provided a variety of solutions to all kinds of domestic and economic problems (Machado 2003).

In addition to the healing by the Holy Ghost, to win converts away from other religions, neo-Pentecostal churches such as the IURD resurrected the exorcism, a technique long familiar in Christianity. Renaming it liberation (*libertação*), they conducted exorcisms not on single individuals but on entire congregations (Lehmann 1996:139–42).

The dramatic centerpiece of an IURD meeting is a collective liberation in which the pastor leads his congregation in expelling spirits once believed in, and perhaps still being received by, many of the visitors and new members who previously had participated in Umbanda, Candomblé, or another Afro-Brazilian group. The Pentecostals consider all the spirits of the other groups to be embodiments of the devil. In a frenzied state, many Umbandistas and participants in other Afro-Spiritist groups who enter trance in response to the singing of evangelical music, clapping of hands, and stomping of feet receive an exu, pomba gira, or other deity. When this happens, uniformed ushers drag the possessed person from his or her seat to the altar, where the pastor takes on the demon, asking it to identify itself. After first refusing, in a practice reminiscent of the Kardecist disobsession (see also Greenfield 2004), it is persuaded by the mystical authority of the pastor. Defeated by the "truth," the demon departs, leaving its human host in a prostrated heap but now liberated—and free to join the IURD. The emotional display often awes those present and leads many of them to immediately accept the Lord (Chestnut 1997:46).

To the miracle healings by the Holy Spirit and the exorcism, Macedo added one more element that had its origins in North America and was critical to his success. In the 1950s, to pay for the increasing costs of television, evangelist Oral Roberts preached a doctrine of prosperity, promising a life of abundance to financial supporters. Other American televangelists elaborated on this idea by promising God's "blessings" to the faithful in the next life and, through baptism in the Holy Spirit, in this world too (Mariano 2003). Macedo made the theology of health and wealth another pillar of the IURD.

"To be blessed by God, as in the Old Testament," writes Cesar (2000:22), referring to the teachings of Macedo and other preachers of the IURD, "means also to have material goods, to become rich. ... Jesus did not want anyone to be sick or poor."

Macedo adopted the "popular" Catholic pattern of the vow, in which fealty is exchanged conditionally for supernatural intercession in attaining the request of a petitioner, but modified it to offer the poverty-stricken urban masses God's blessings in exchange for their first accepting the Holy Ghost. Being baptized in the IURD, new members agreed to serve God, which in accepted Christian tradition meant paying a tithe. "Contrary to the 'promises' made by Catholics when the believer pays for what he or she received" (Cesar 2000:30), the members of the IURD are told to pay God first. Doing so, Macedo claims, makes God indebted to them and obligated to provide whatever they may ask him for. Should a prayer not be answered, Macedo tells the disappointed member of the congregation, he or she does not have sufficient faith and must petition God harder—which is to say, increase the value of his or her offering to the church.

The IURD used the massive amounts of money given by its millions of members to purchase not just television stations but all forms of media and other enterprises. According to Fonseca (2003:259; see also Mariano 2003), the church corporation has sixty-two radio stations (twenty-one AM and thirty-one FM) and sixty-three television stations that bring its message to 85 percent of Brazil's major cities and into three hundred municipalities. It publishes its own newspaper, the *Folha Universal,* with a circulation of 1.5 million, and a secular paper, the *Hoje em Dia* of Belo Horizonte. It owns a publishing company that has produced thirty-four books by Edir Macedo, plus a recording firm that by the year 2000 had title to more than 900,000 CDs. Its partial list of assets in Brazil includes construction, data processing, video, travel, and consulting companies. Overseas, it has holdings in the Cayman and Channel islands (Mariano 2003:238–39). In the 1990s it transformed what had been an indebtedness of $45 million in its media holdings into a $300 million positive balance. Macedo, in the image of the Pentecostals described by Curry, created a veritable feitoria—a factory of twenty-first century enterprises that produce wealth in amounts only imagined by Brazil's early sugar and coffee barons.

The key to the success Macedo and his fellow neo-Pentecostals have had in attracting new members is healing. In exchange for being cured by the Holy Ghost, the Pentecostal variant of the supernatural, Brazilians in need convert, as do others who are helped by the spirits of their competitors. Now, as participants in an evangelical denomination, they engage in its rituals and enthusiastically bring its truth to the world.

CHAPTER 13

HEALING IN THE COMPETITIVE RELIGIOUS MARKETPLACE

Had Celestina de Araujo Santos, the young woman who became an Umbanda medium, not obtained relief from back pains and other problems, she certainly would not have returned to the Casa de Vovô Maria and completed the exchange that resulted in her becoming an adept. But her quest for assistance would not have ended, for it is unlikely that she would have resigned herself to the discomfort and suffering. Unlike the average North American, she may not have gone from one doctor or medical clinic to another. Instead, more likely, she would have confided her problems to another relative, friend, coworker, or mere acquaintance, and this discussion would have led her to one of the other competing religious groups. "There is not one Brazilian," writes St. Clair (1971:237), "who doesn't have a 'spirit story' to tell, be it something that happened personally or else to a friend or a member of the family." Let us suppose that she was directed to a Spiritist healer-medium, the head of one of the "more African" religious centers, or perhaps an evangelical church. Had she spoken with someone who previously was successful with Spiritism, the spirit of a deceased doctor such as Fritz or Stams, incorporated in the body of an Edson Queiroz, Mauricio Magalhães, or Antonio de Oliveira Rios, might have helped her. During this treatment, the young beautician might have been told that she had mediumistic ability that should be developed. The implicit exchange between the sufferer and this view of the world of the supernatural is that if healed, the sufferer is obligated, as payment for what was received, to learn the Kardecist ritual practices and to receive its spirits and help others in need as part of the tradition's mission of charity. Instead of becoming an Umbandista after being helped by the preto velho, Celestina would have become a Kardecist.

Should she have spoken to a member of a Candomblé terreiro she might have sought the assistance of the orixá that was divined to be the "owner of her head." And had the ritual treatment proposed by the mãe- or pai-de-santo been followed and been successful, the beautician instead would have been committed to an initiatory training program during which she would have learned to provide for her deities, who in turn (or in exchange) would heal and continue to care for her. In brief, in exchange for the help received, Celestina could have become an active member of a Candomblé, a Xangô, a Macumba, or a Batuque terreiro. And had she chanced to speak first to someone who participated in one of the many evangelical Protestant groups, or heard on the radio or seen on television one of their ubiquitous testimonials, which tell of the presenter being helped by the Holy Spirit, her trajectory could have been that taken by Creuza, one of Cecília Mariz's (1994:38) informants.

Creuza, humiliated and desperate after her husband was unable to find work and after she took sick, leaving their children destitute, made a vow to the God of the crentes. Creuza promised that if he gave a job to her husband, enabled her to get food for her family without begging, and cured her, she would become a believer. When her husband almost immediately found work and she recovered her health, Crueza joined the Pentecostal Church.[31] And as Chestnut generalizes, evoking a Pentecostal analogy with Maria da Fatima Batista's pilgrimage experience: "Reflecting the clientelism that continues to characterize Brazilian social, political, and religious relationships, the Holy Spirit operates as a sort of divine patron, offering protection in exchange for service and loyalty" (1997:96).

In what is almost commonplace in Brazil, Celestina might have gone from one (competing) religious group to the next, offering a commitment to its specific form of devotional practice in return for assistance. Unlike the era prior to the end of Catholic hegemony, when most inhabitants of Brazil lived in rural areas and knew only of the Catholic saints—or the African orixás, syncretized or not— urban residents today have available to them a range of supernatural beings, each provided by a competing faith, to whom they may offer devotion and affiliation in exchange for help with their numerous problems. To adequately understand the broader setting within which individual Brazilians are making choices that result in bargains with the supernatural in their search for assistance with health-related and other problems, some background on the transformation and growth that occurred in the population and economy of Brazilian society in the second half of the twentieth century is required.

In 1940 the country's population was slightly more than 41 million, up considerably from a little over 18 million at the beginning of the twentieth century. Twenty-six percent, or approximately 10 million people, lived in urban centers, including eleven cities with populations of more than 200,000. A decade later, the national census counted 10 million more people, 8 million of whom were in cities of more than 200,000. One-third of all Brazilians were now classified as city dwellers, with the remaining two-thirds residing in the rural hinterland (Santos 1993:29).

In the 1950s the federal government put in place new economic policies that favored import substitution, industrialization, and disinvestments in the rural, agricultural sector. The consequent decline in agriculture led millions of displaced workers, no longer needed by landowners, to relocate from the interior to cities where new factories were being built. Since Brazilian industrialization was capital rather than labor intensive, from the beginning jobs were not created to sufficiently absorb the ever-expanding population arriving regularly in search of work. Moreover, only a tiny fraction of the immigrants from the interior had the skills required to obtain employment. Jobs in other sectors of the economy also did not grow in proportion to the numbers of people added to the labor force each year. Brazil's fast-growing cities came to be the home of large numbers of unemployed and underemployed.

When the national population increased to 70 million in 1960, those in cities had grown to 32 million, 45 percent of the total. In the next two decades the number of people in Brazil exploded, reaching 119 million in 1980, with 82 million of them, or 69 percent, living in cities. Fifty million people had been added to the nation's urban centers, while the rural population remained stable at 38 million. In ten cities, the population exceeded more than one million inhabitants, with Rio de Janeiro at 9 million and São Paulo at more than 12.5 million (Santos 1993:86).

In 1990 more than 80 percent of the nation's 150 million people resided in major metropolitan centers—more than 100 million more people than had been living in cities in 1940. In the last two decades of the twentieth century, the number of Brazilians continued to expand, reaching 180 million by 2000, ten times greater than the population at the opening of the century. With minor exceptions, the vast majority of Brazilians were located within 100 miles of the Atlantic coast.

In the early years of industrialization, workers fortunate enough to find employment joined unions and obtained job security and health, retirement, and other benefits. After privatization in the 1990s, in response to the worldwide process of globalization driven by the free market policies of the World Bank and the International Monetary Fund, decisions about production, finance, and employment practices suddenly were made by transnational corporations located thousands of miles away. These multinational corporations did not have a stake in, or care about the consequences of their actions for, Brazilian society or its people. Downsizing became the order of the day. The restructuring of the world economy exacerbated this depressing situation. Jobs in the industrial sector were outsourced, with workers now given short-term contracts without protection or benefits. Real wages, in industry and agriculture, continue to decline. The minimum wage, despite being raised, decreased in purchasing power. Today, a growing percentage of Brazilians are finding it difficult to support themselves and their families.

One way to conceptualize the extent of the poverty prevailing currently in Brazil is in terms of the inequality in the distribution of wealth and national income. While there have been significant disparities between rich and the poor in the nation since colonial times, the inequality has become far greater with industrialization, urbanization, and globalization. In 2007 the minimum wage, earned by approximately 32 percent of the workforce, was raised to R$380 per month, up from R$300 in 2005 and R$260 in 2004.[32] It would take R$864.59 per month, however, to regain the buying power of the minimum wage of the year 1940, when it was introduced (Fleischer, December 11–17, 2004), and R$1,924.59 to sustain a family of four adequately today (Star Online 2008). In 2003 53.9 million Brazilians were classified as poor, according to the Instituto de Pesquisa Econômica Aplicada (Institute for Applied Economic Research IPEA), with 21.9 million of them as indigent (Fleischer, March 27–April 1, 2005). In 2004, according to the Instituto Brasileira de Geografia e Estatística (IBGE), the national statistics service, 44.8 million Brazilians lived below the "misery line" (Fleischer, November 26–December 2, 2005). Some 6.6 million lived in favelas, or squatter settlements, and 41.8 million did not have access to clean water, sewers, or trash collection. The officially accepted unemployment rate, believed by critics to be significantly understated, has hovered around 10 percent in recent years.[33] At the end of 2005, there were 1.4 million unemployed in Brazil's largest cities, 44.5 percent of them between the ages of sixteen and twenty-four (Fleischer, September 9–15, 2006). Brazil's Gini Index, which measures income (and other concentrations of wealth) and ranges from 0 (no concentrations) to 1.00 (total inequality), was 0.86 in 2005 (Fleischer, January 12–18, 2008). This index confirms what most of Brazil's religious leaders have known and is painfully experienced by the majority of those to whom they appeal.

Brazil is frequently acknowledged to be one of the most (economically) unjust nations in the world. In 1995 a fifth of the population, or 32 million people, received only 2.5 percent of the national income. The lowest 40 percent received slightly more than 8 percent of the total and the poorest half only one-tenth of it. The highest quintile, meanwhile, received 64.2 percent of the national income. National income going to the lowest half of the population dropped from 17.4 percent in the 1960s to 12.6 percent in 1980 and continued to decline to the end of the century (Saboia, quoted in Corten 1999:104). [34] Since the poorest 10 percent of Brazilian wage earners have a tax burden equivalent to 32.8 percent of their income, compared to only 22.7 percent for the richest 10 percent (Fleischer, May 10–16, 2008), the chances of them catching up seem remote. Moreover, although inflation has been generally under control since the end of the twentieth century, for purchases, it was almost 3 percent higher on an annual basis (for 2008) for low-income earners (between 1 and 2.5 minimum wages) than for those with incomes considerably higher (Fleischer, May 10–16, 2008). Twenty seven million children presently live below the poverty line in families that earn less than $R4.33 a day (*Brazilians* 2004–05:10, citing a UNICEF report). The UN's Millennium Project, launched in 2002, identified thirteen "pockets of poverty" in Brazil that included 26 million inhabitants in 600 municípios (municipalities), with Human Development Index (HDI) scores on a par with Uganda (Fleischer, January 15–21, 2005). The president of the Inter-American Development Bank said that to eliminate poverty and make Brazilian society "just" may take as long as a century.

Brazil's cities were not prepared for the massive influx of rural migrants during the second half of the twentieth century, nor did they provide the infrastructure to accommodate them. Since there were not enough dwellings to house the population, vast and continuously growing numbers came to live in favelas located at the margins of urban centers. Favelas appeared on hillsides, swamplands, and the urban outskirts that were not considered habitable by people of substance. Energy sources, means of transportation, telephone lines, water, and sewage were inadequate. Inevitable results were endemic and chronic diseases such as cholera, dengue fever, meningitis, and viral and bacterial infections. Alcoholism, drugs, prostitution, gambling, gangs, and gang warfare flourished, further complicating the insecurity and dangers confronting the population.

Now, in spite of more than half a century of national experience with, and debate over, the conditions of hunger, illness, and poverty, they are still conceptualized and treated as the problems of the sufferer. In exchange for votes, politicians at first took the lead in presenting themselves as the ones best able to assist the growing population. When the political process was unable to cope with, or provide satisfaction to, those in need, the popular or alternative religious groups stepped in. They attracted converts by focusing on alleviating the physical, mental, and emotional suffering of the urban masses, much of which manifested itself in illness and unease.

Each encounter with a new religion and its supernatural(s) presents an opportunity for the resolution of a specific problem by someone in need. Should a person making a request cease experiencing the symptoms that precipitated the quest, he or she reciprocates the gift received and converts to a new religion by performing its acts of ritual and devotion. But, as we have seen, the treatments of each group do not work for all individuals on all occasions. Edson Queiroz/Dr. Fritz might remove a growth on Fatima's shoulder without pain and complications today, but the same positive outcome may not occur should she return with back pains, debilitating headaches, or a malignant tumor some weeks or months or years later. St. Francis might have cured a pilgrim paying his debt today, but there is no guarantee that another miracle will occur for that individual in the future. So the ailing party might seek help from one of the other groups, praying or going to public sessions and receiving treatment at one center or church or another, seeking the help of the supernatural through intermediaries.

The implication of this situation is that although Celestina and Marco Antônio became Umbandistas in exchange for help from Umbanda spirits, Fatima and Dona Clarice went back to the Catholic Church when St. Francis interceded on their behalf, and others became members of Candomblé terreiros, Spiritist centers, or evangelical churches as payment for the help of their supernatural(s), their conversion must be seen as a temporary phenomenon. While Dr. Fritz or the leaders of the several competing religious groups may be convinced that exposure to spectacular cures that defy common sense will bring them converts, they neglect the fact that they do not cure everyone all the time. The result is that Brazilians trek from one religious group to the next until they obtain what they request, but once they convert, there is no guarantee they will remain loyal. Should their next crisis not be resolved by the spirits of the group whose rituals they practice, they will turn to another group and still other until satisfaction is eventually obtained. Consequently, the average Brazilian may become a member of several religions over the course of a lifetime, giving us at the sociological level a pattern of individuals moving, or circulating, from religion to religion over time.[35] Hence the number of members that each religious group can honestly claim will vary, with considerable overlap, since members at any time may be in the process of changing their affiliation.[36]

PART II. HEALING BY THE SPIRITS IN OTHER BRAZILIAN RELIGIONS

This analysis does not negate Dr. Fritz's challenge. How do we explain the spectacular acts of healing described in the preceding chapters? Did the supernatural entities, be they spirits like Drs. Fritz and Stams, saints such as Francis, the Holy Ghost of the Pentecostals, the African orixás of the Candomblés and Batuques, or the pretos velhos and pomba giras of Umbanda, really heal the millions who claim they did? The dilemma posed by Dr. Fritz remains. If the healings performed and described defy our commonsense understandings in that they cannot be explained in terms of medicine, or other sciences as we know them, must we accept Fritz's claim that the healings are to be attributed to spirits? And if so, and we are to be rational, are we required, as Fritz claims, to accept Kardecist-Spiritism as the belief system to replace science? Furthermore, since the other religions of Brazil and elsewhere also offer therapeutic treatments—based on a belief in their supernatural beings—that result in cures not unlike those of their Kardecist competitors, must we then choose among them? Is the only alternative to the inability of medical science to explain surgeries without anesthesia and antisepsis, and the equally inexplicable recoveries, to cast aside science and return to religion?

Before the reader feels the need to choose between the competing appeals of the contending parties in the religious marketplace in Brazil, let me raise a broader question that I will attempt to answer in the final section of this volume from the perspective of a skeptical scientist: Is it possible that supernatural entities really can heal? Or put in another way: Can a belief in a specific supernatural and its ability to help contribute to the healing of patients? And can this be understood within the framework of the sciences that inform modern medicine? We turn to these issues in part III, beginning with the relationship between science and the supernatural.

PART III

SPIRITS, HEALING, AND A NEW PARADIGM

CHAPTER 14

HEALING BY SPIRITS AND SCIENCE

In the late 1950s, as Henry Belk and Andre Puharich drove from São Paulo to Congonhas do Campo in the state of Minas Gerais to meet the already well-known Spiritist medium Zé Arigó for the first time, Puharich, who recently had completed training in medicine, turned to Belk and asked almost whimsically, "Henry, what if it's real?" Neither the medicine he had studied nor the sciences in which that medicine was grounded could explain what they, this author, and so many others were to observe that day and in the years following. Puharich and Belk were to look to parapsychology in their lifelong search for alternative explanations of the unusual events they experienced.

Parapsychology, "the study of the unusual in psychology," focuses on what are called psi phenomena. According to Atkinson, Atkinson, Smith, and Bem (1990:234), these are "processes of information and/or energy not currently explicable in terms of known science." Extrasensory perception (ESP)—which subsumes telepathy, clairvoyance, and precognition—and psychokinesis (PK) are topics of study under parapsychology.

The Greek prefix *para* means "above," "beyond," or "other." Thus *paranormal* refers to things, events, or phenomena that are "above the normal," "beyond the common," "other than the usual," or simply unusual. There are degrees of unusualness, of course. Paranormal seems to be reserved for those phenomena that are *most unusual*—so unusual that they are said to be anomalous: unable to be explained by science, or at least by science as it is known at present.

Calling unusual phenomena paranormal, as Bonewits ([1971] 1993:34) observed, is a "sneaky way" to get around calling them supernatural—or miraculous—and neither psychologists nor parapsychologists have had much interest in the supernatural. (On the category of supernatural, see Greenfield 2003:151–58; Lohmann 2003.)

Dr. Fritz, or the leader of one of the other Brazilian religious groups, could have offered another interpretation of the question Dr. Puharich put to his traveling companion. Did the facts—that the mediums performed surgery without anesthesia and antisepsis, that the patients did not feel pain or develop complications, and that the patients recovered—mean that the spirits were real? When faced with reports of spirits of deceased human beings curing the sick or helping the living, how is the scientifically oriented scholar to think, understand, and write about them?

Anthropologist Morton Klass (1995:28) grappled with this question in a chapter called "The Problem with Supernatural" in a book attempting to define religion. He began by presenting the case of a Trinidadian villager, commonly referred to at the time of the research as of East Indian descent, who left an offering of the blood of a cockerel (a small fowl), an oil lamp, some flowers, and a cigarette to the spirit of the field in gratitude for a good rice harvest. The problem, as Klass notes, was not with the villager but rather with our own recognition of, and the opposition we make between, the categories (or domains) of the natural and the supernatural. Klass concludes, following John Beattie, "The trouble with such distinctions is that very often [researchers] commit the cardinal sin of social anthropology, by imputing to another culture a kind of category-making which is characteristic of our own practically oriented, 'scientistic' society" (Klass 1995:31, citing Beattie 1964:203). "The only solution," Klass continues, "at least as far as I can see, is to give up, once and for all the effort to maintain this dubious dichotomy." "The dichotomizing of natural as against supernatural," he concludes, "remains invincibly ethnocentric and therefore unsuitable for anthropological analysis" (Klass 1995:32).

Chapter 14. Healing by Spirits and Science

Sir Edward B. Tylor, a founding father of anthropology, and Sir James Frazer, a prominent early student of comparative religion, both employed this dichotomy and in doing so deprecated the beliefs of the mostly poor and unsophisticated informants who claimed, like those reported on here, to have been cured by spirits. Frazer was very clear when he wrote that religious leaders, whom he refers to as sorcerers and magicians, "were in principle all alike, they were for the most part charlatans living off the gullibility of their clients." He added, "*It must always be remembered that every single profession and claim put forward by the magician as such is false; not one of them can be maintained without deception, conscious or unconscious*" (Klass 1995:72–73, citing Frazer [1911–15] 1922:53; italics added by Klass).

And since there is no truth in any of it, which is to say that it has never and cannot happen, Frazer concluded, "I hope that after this explicit disclaimer I shall no longer be taxed with embracing a system of mythology which I look upon not merely as false but as preposterous and absurd" (quoted in Klass 1995:1).

Frazer and Tylor were not the only anthropologists, and certainly not the only Western scholars and students of religion, to feel obliged to distance themselves from the beliefs and practices of those whose ways of life they reported on by telling their readers that it was not really so. Franz Boas (1966:121) and W. Bogaras ([1904–09] 1979:302), who worked in the tradition of science, responded similarly. In a case reported in the New York Times, medical researchers who found that Korean women in an in vitro fertilization clinic who were prayed for, without being told, had higher pregnancy rates than those who were not prayed for "thought long and hard about whether to publish their findings, since they seemed so improbable" (Nagourney 2001). On a personal level, I can add the reaction of an anonymous reviewer of a manuscript describing surgeries attributed to Dr. Fritz and other spirits that I submitted to an anthropology journal. The commentator recommended not publishing the article, not because of its substance but rather because the reviewer simply did not believe that patients operated on in this way did not feel pain or develop infections. It was all too improbable. This stance goes back to the beginnings of science and its effort to separate itself from religion.

What Copernicus, Kepler, Galileo, Newton, and other founders of modern science successfully challenged when they proposed an alternative explanation for the movement of the planets was not religion, as the oversimplified version in most textbooks tells us, but rather a given set of assumptions about how the world worked that was rooted in the Christianity of the period. This view of the world, as championed by the then hegemonic Roman Catholic Church (and still championed by its popular variant, as expressed in pilgrimages, and other competing groups in Brazil's religious marketplace), rested on the acceptance of a supernatural who intervened regularly in the workings of the universe he was believed to have created. It was the will of this all-powerful being that was purported to explain everything, from the movement of the planets to the behavior of human beings, including their suffering from, or being cured of, illnesses.

Science refuted neither God's existence nor his having made the universe but instead offered an alternative. The former single reality that had encompassed everything was partitioned into two distinct and separate realms. The natural was allocated to science for study and explanation. The supernatural remained the realm of God, who, from the perspective of the science of the period, was reconceptualized so as to retain a relationship to the natural world. God became the master architect and mathematician who designed the material world in the image of a complex machine, from which he stepped back, leaving it to run according to his design.

René Descartes ([1637, 1641] 1980) provided the philosophical foundation and guiding imagery by which science, understood as the project to discover the assumed order (or laws) in the (natural) universe, imposed by the creator, was to be carried out. Skeptical of all forms of knowledge, he argued that *res cognitas*—"thinking substance, subjective experience, spirit, consciousness, that which man perceives as within—was understood as fundamentally different and separate from *res extensa*—extended substance, the objective world, matter, the physical body, plants and animals, stones and stars, the entire physical universe. . . . Only in man did the two realities come together as mind and body" (Tarnas 1991:278).

"Hence," as Tarnas continues, "on the one side of Descartes' dualism soul and the spiritual [including the supernatural], is understood as mind, and human awareness as distinctively that of the thinker. … On the other side of the dualism, and in contrast to the mind, all objects of the external world lack subjective awareness, purpose or spirit" (1991:278).

In this imagery, which became the basis of early modern science, the investigator used only his critical reason to discover the order in what was assumed to be an objective material universe. All else that was mind, and part of the human potential to create belief systems and views of the world, was to be covered over and held in abeyance. That which was being studied was assumed to be nothing other than an inert substance whose workings were determined by an invariant set of rules external to it.[37] With respect to what was classified as the supernatural, the Cartesian framework placed it outside the natural world, making it impossible for it on a priori grounds to interfere with or influence anything in what was referred to as the "real" world. Cartesian science excluded whatever was placed in the category supernatural from scientific examination. No wonder those who claimed to be scientists or (Western) educated individuals schooled in scientific thought were unable to consider, even for discussion, anything that as much as suggested the possible intervention of something from the supernatural category in the material world.

Descartes' dualism had perhaps its greatest influence in the development of medicine, in terms of which the surgeries and healings discussed previously are inexplicable. Consistent with early science in general, medicine took as its province the res extensas phenomenon that for it was the material human body. A black box was placed over res cognitas, the mind of the human organism. Only in this way could medicine proceed to treat a sick person as if he or she were a machine composed of a series of interrelated parts, which could be manipulated like a motor, independent of the surrounding environment of feelings, beliefs, and emotions of the organism—that is, his or her mind:

> The body could be regarded as a separate "thing" outside the patient's self. Surgical intervention in particular seemed to require that the body, at least temporarily, be removed from spiritual or personal meanings. (Osherson and AmaraSingham 1981:226)

Medical treatment consequently was free to develop along the lines of machine repair. If a body did not work, parts were fixed or changed with surgery or, alternatively, pharmaceuticals were administered to repair the damage and restore the body to its "normal" functioning state. When science eventually began to examine that aspect of the human organism over which the followers of Cartesian science had placed the proverbial black box, the mind was not refor-mulated as res cognitas.[38]

Within the science of medicine, the mind—first thought of as that which ran the machine—was allocated to the new science of psychology. The implication of this allocation for the purpose of my analysis is that all the rest of res cognitas came to be attributes of the minds of human beings taken one at a time. The social and cultural dimensions just beginning at the time to be studied by the disciplines of sociology and anthropology are only now being intro-duced into discussions of mind/body interrelations. Not only does something approaching a paradigm shift seem to be required to add what has been learned from psychology to ameliorate the restric-tive implications of the dualism that divorced body from mind in science's approach to medicine and healing, but a second one might be required to ameliorate the individualizing and psychologizing of mind to bring back the remainder of res cognitas, including the supernatural.

How can this be done? Given that scientific thinking, and spe-cifically for our purposes the paradigm of medical science as it is currently taught and practiced, is based on the natural/supernatu-ral dichotomy and the body/mind dualism, in which the latter term means the psychological attributes of the individual, how would we proceed were we to accept Klass's suggestion that anthropolo-gists and other Western scholars give up the natural/supernatural dichotomy?

Psychologist Lawrence LeShan (1995) has offered a possible solu-tion to the problem of how to integrate the supernatural into the framework of science. In his analysis of Uvani, the "spirit control" of the American medium Eileen Garrett (the spirit said to orient her, much like Drs. Fritz and Stam, the orixás, pretos velhos, pomba giras, Holy Ghost Pentecostal converts, and Catholic saints ori-ent their followers), he asks the question: *When* is Uvani? From the perspective of scientific analysis, he proposes that spirit beings be thought of as functional as opposed to structural concepts. Struc-tural concepts, he contends, "are things with length, breadth, and thickness" (LeShan 1995:167). They have a definite physical exis-tence and continue with this existence whether or not they are at a particular moment in anyone's consciousness.

Functional entities, in contrast,

> do not have any length, breadth, or thickness. They cannot be detected by any form of instrumentation, although their effects often can be. ...They do not have continuous existence whether or not they are being mentally conceptualized ... they exist only when they are held in a mind, only when being conceptualized, only when being considered to exist. (LeShan 1995:167)

As an example of a functional concept, LeShan suggests the useful mathematical device the square root of minus one. "One would be hard put—or find it impossible—to solve many mathematical or engineering problems without it" (LeShan 1995:168). But there is no such number as the square root of minus one. It does not exist independent of the conscious agreement of members of the mathematical community. It was invented to help explain things that otherwise could not have been understood. It is not relevant that unlike structural concepts used in mathematics it is *not real.*

Another example of a functional entity or concept offered by LeShan is gravity,[39] which "is a very useful one and enables us to explain old data and to predict new data, but its characteristics are explained by saying that those are its characteristics" (LeShan 1995:171). Independent of the agreement of students of the physical order, it does not exist. A functional entity, therefore, is what we agree it is and/or does and when it does it.

Are we then to take this to mean that spirits and the supernatural are what we agree they are based on what they do and when they do it? This is how most concepts used to describe and analyze culture are formulated. Anthropologist might agree, but would physicians and others trained in medicine and its healing practices? Since there is no place for the supernatural in the way science is conceptualized in psychology, most psychologists would reject such a formulation. Do we have to forgo being scientists if we wish to deal with the supernatural? If so, must we then adopt the epistemologies and classificatory systems of our informants? In the case of the surgeries and other therapeutic interventions being discussed here, is there an alternative to accepting Dr. Fritz's claim, or those of his rivals? Or must we go back to the extant beliefs prevailing in the West prior to the advent of science?

It seems to me that a solution such as Klass proposes would enable us to report and analyze the beliefs and classificatory systems of our informants, but only as distinct and independent forms of thought. Comparison and contrast between any one belief system and our own or another might be possible, if we choose to push the postmodernist envelope. But would there be a way to translate from one system into another, such as from that of a small, still partially isolated population marginal to the Western world to the generally held understandings of our academic colleagues and Western-educated readers? At this point, it seems unlikely that it would be possible to translate what we learn from others into scientific thought. To resolve this dilemma, I propose returning to the foundations of scientific thought and to the metaphor on which the Cartesian dualism is based to see if we can reconceptualize it so as to replace or bring together the oppositional dualism of natural/supernatural and body/mind, along with the almost exclusive use of individual psychology, in the understanding of the mind, to introduce aspects of the social and cultural into a reformulation of science and its applications in healing.

Such a reformulation is already underway by scholars attempting to include the role of the mind in the healing process. While many of these thinkers would probably bristle at the introduction of the supernatural and other aspects of culture into the framework they are developing, I propose to show that doing so in terms of their efforts at reconceptualization will add to their undertaking while offering a framework for understanding and explaining the healing experienced by the Brazilians discussed above.

The next chapter provides a brief epistemological summary of the nature of scientific thought, after which I turn to the reformulation of the body/mind dichotomy and reintroduce the supernatural as an aspect of culture.

CHAPTER 15

SCIENCE AS A CULTURAL PROCESS

In his classic study *The Structure of Scientific Revolutions*, the late Thomas Kuhn (1970:3–4) asks how someone ignorant of the history of science would examine electrical or chemical (or other) phenomena if inclined to do so. "What must the world be like," he queries in his closing argument, "in order that man may know it?"

To anthropologists, the answer is found in symbolism. That is, it calls for the formulation of a mental picture, expressible in words that order representations of what the world is like. Alternative images are possible. The specifics of any one image selected serve as the building blocks on which an understanding of the chemical, electrical, or other phenomena can be developed. Since people other than scientists are curious about the world around them, they too must develop a mental picture or symbolic model that will enable them to explore, analyze, and eventually gain an understanding of the events they experience and the phenomena they encounter. Science, as we have become increasingly aware, is a cultural process. Acknowledging this enables us to treat the doing of science as comparable to, and illustrative of, our understanding of other forms of cultural practice. Furthermore, it enables us to separate persons seeking to understand the world into two categories: 1) scientists and scholars; 2) at least some of those they study (Greenfield and Droogers 2003:32).

To satisfy their curiosity about aspects of the world they encounter, actors in both categories develop models that, when elaborated and tested over time, form a basis for understanding. Occasionally, the scientist, more specifically the social scientist, and the people studied find themselves interested in the same events or phenomena. The images, models, and theories of the scientist may or may not overlap or be congruent with those of the people studied.

The simplest answer to Kuhn's "what must the world be like" question is to be found in metaphor (see D'Andrade 1995; Quinn 1991; Fernandez 1991, 1986; Quinn and Holland 1987). By likening the world to something already known, the curious person (scientist or layperson) may use what knowledge he or she has about the known to think about the unknown and formulate questions about it. The answers to the questions provide further insights and understandings that may be explored in detail.

Kuhn reminds us that effective research

> scarcely begins before a scientific community thinks it has acquired firm answers to questions like the following: What are the fundamental entities of which the universe is composed? How do these interact with each other and with the senses? What questions may legitimately be asked about the entities and what techniques employed in seeking solutions? (1970:4–5)

Kuhn acknowledges that far from being absolute, the answers are arbitrary. They derive from the particular image of what the world is like adopted by members of a scientific community.

Kuhn then does something that shows keen anthropological insight. He moves from his initial discussion of an isolated individual asking about natural phenomena to a scientific community. Such a community is a social group formed around a shared image of what the world is like and how one studies it. The consensus its members hold enables them to ask similar questions, the answers to which expand their collective understanding of their field or subject of interest.

Once a paradigm, defined as "an accepted model or pattern," is agreed upon, the individual members do "puzzle solving," posing questions, the hypothesized answers to which can be tested (Kuhn 1970:23). This process requires agreement by members of a scientific community as to the terms, referred to as concepts, that enable them to relate observed events or data to the conceptual categories of their paradigm.

Taken cumulatively, the answers to the many questions asked and puzzles solved fill in the blanks or unknowns in the paradigm or model. This in turn expands the scientific community's knowledge of what the world is like and hence its ability to explain the phenomena of interest to it.

Before proceeding, two points in Kuhn's presentation are worth emphasizing. First, the questions asked by scientists and scholars are not about some absolute reality but rather are derived from, and are the products of, the specific model or paradigm around which a consensus has developed. Independent of a shared mental picture, concepts, and the hypotheses they are used to formulate, have neither meaning nor relevance.

Secondly, techniques used to solve the puzzles and methods employed by members of a scientific community to test and validate theories are based on and derived from the images of their shared paradigm or model. In Kuhn's words: "The existence of the paradigm sets the problem to be solved; often the paradigm theory is implicated directly in the design of the apparatus able to solve the problem" (Kuhn 1970:27).

Not all puzzles can be solved. Occasionally scientists encounter anomalies that cannot be explained in terms of their agreed-on paradigm, such as those posed by the Spiritist surgeries and other controversial therapies reported here. If the anomalies are of a sufficient magnitude, they may bring the utility of the paradigm itself into question. With the consensus shattered, members of the scientific community may propose an alternative image as to what the world is like that ideally will incorporate previous knowledge while making it possible to account for the anomalies.

In the natural sciences, where a single paradigm had tended to dominate studies of particular subject matters or disciplines, the proposal of a new imagery to deal with anomalies in any one invariably led to conflict between members of the scientific community. This process of paradigm replacement is the "scientific revolution" referred to in Kuhn's title.

The paradigm that informed the medical sciences and provided our commonsense standards of "reality" with respect to healing was based on the Cartesian mind/body opposition. It led us and our medical professionals to treat the body as *if* it were a machine. Based on this mechanical imagery, a doctor might be likened to a mechanic who repairs or replaces parts of, or introduces materials into, human bodies in an effort to get them to retain or return to optimal operating efficiency. Once the imagery was accepted as the paradigm for treating the sick, it was possible for researchers to zero in on specific problems—solving puzzles in Kuhn's terms. The thousands of hypotheses, experiments, theories, and research trials analyzed statistically and reported regularly in the scientific literature and the popular press exemplify how scientists have tried to solve puzzles. Some seemed not to be solvable, meaning that certain forms of suffering—whether or not classified as illnesses—continued to afflict patients, while some treatments that led to cures could not be explained in terms of the paradigm. The anomalies, corroborating Kuhn's view of paradigm shifts, led individuals to search for other imageries, or ways to modify the prevailing one, that might explain the anomalies, thus resulting in the modification or transformation of the predominant framework. The direction this change took emphasized process, transformation, and interrelatedness and not the stasis of the mechanical model.

By the end of the nineteenth century, the absolutes of space, time, object, and determinism were apparently securely enthroned in an unmysterious, mechanically determined world, basically simple in structure at the atomic level and, statistically at least, unchanging in form—for even geological and biological transformations operated under fixed laws (Peacocke 1979:54).

In the early years of the twentieth century, as McFague summarized it, "there was a movement toward a model more aptly described as organic, for there occurred a profound realization of the deep relations between space, time, and matter, which relativized them all. ... [R]elationships and relativity as well as processes and openness, characterize reality as it is understood at present in all branches of science" (1987:10).

Chance and necessity replace determinism in this new picture. Individuals always exist within structures of relationship. Process, change, transformation, and openness replace stasis. Interdependence, novelty, and even mystery are part of the new understanding of reality (McFague 1987:10). In this imagery, one does not "enter into relations" with others, as McFague informs us, "but finds oneself in such relationships as the most basic given of existence" (1987:11). In the mechanistic model, entities are separated dualistically and hierarchically, while in the organic, or "mutualistic" one, all entities are considered to be subjects as well as objects. A key element is their communication with each other and the interaction it makes possible. This thinking is at the forefront of anthropology and the newly expanding fields of medicine such as immunology, endocrinology, neurology, and psychoneuroimmunology. Researchers have questioned the Cartesian mind/body dualism and are replacing it with a framework of interrelatedness and information flow to integrate the biophysiological, mental, and emotional dimensions of being human into the understanding of illness and its treatment.

CHAPTER 16

COMMUNICATION, INFORMATION FLOW, AND A NEW PARADIGM

There are many ... instances in the history of science where important information does not make an impact at the time of its discovery, but lies "dormant" until inspired creative insight reveals its true worth.

Steele, Lindley, and Blanden 1998

The outline of what I am proposing as a new imagery for the healing sciences, which will provide a model for understanding the unusual data presented in parts 1 and 2, is to be found on parallel and still unconnecting tracks at the opposite extremes of the body/mind divide. On the side of the mind, medical anthropology offers a model of symbolic transformation where in response to a flow of information at the cultural level, usually while participating in a social ritual, an afflicted individual undergoes a transformation that results in the abatement or disappearance of debilitating symptoms. The process is referred to as embodiment. The suffering person receives the information provided in the therapeutic ritual, and this leads to recovery. Thus far, no attempts to ask how this works have been made. What happens in the body in response to the information in the ritual that precipitates the transformation?

On the other side of the dualism, in a groundbreaking series of experiments, neurobiologist Candace Pert and her colleagues (Pert 1997; Pert et al. 1985), and others, demonstrated how information flows through the body, carried by chemical molecules that lock on to receptors on the cells. Moreover, they also showed that brain function is modulated by the flow of chemicals.[40] In brief, body and mind, conceptualized as brain, were integrated, with their component parts interacting within a single system.

Psychologist Ernest L. Rossi ([1986] 1993; see also Rossi and Rossi 1996) took the next step in a brilliant book, *The Psychobiology of Mind-Body Healing*, in which he formulated an information/communication model that related important breakthroughs in psychotherapy and hypnotherapy to propose the new vision of brain/body information flow.

Following Black, who first suggested "how hypnosis could modulate psychophysiological mechanisms of the immune system" (quoted in Rossi [1986] 1993:26–27; cf. Black 1969), Rossi cites Bowers, not just in proposing the flow of information as an imagery for rethinking the relationship between mind and body but also in suggesting a mechanism for the interrelationship and interaction between what previously had been thought of as separate and distinct systems, composed of subsystems called body and mind.

> The entire human body can be viewed as an interlocking network of informational systems—genetic, immunological, hormonal, and so on. These systems each have their own codes, and transmission of information between systems requires some sort of transducer that allows the code of one system, genetic, say, to be translated into the code of another system—for example, immunological.
>
> Now, the mind, with its capacity for symbolizing in linguistic and extra-linguistic forms, can also be regarded as a means for coding, processing and transmitting information both intra- and inter-personality. If information processing and transmission is common to both psyche and soma, the mind-body problem might be reformulated as follows: How is information, received and processed at the semantic level, transduced into information that can be received and processed at the somatic level, and vice-versa? That sounds like a question that can be more sensibly addressed than the one it is meant to replace. (Bowers 1977:231; quoted in Rossi 1993:27)

The idea that information may flow between different systems within a complex organism, or separate systems at different levels, is basic to the new way of thinking. That it is decipherable in terms of a code and, if transduced,[41] may be integrated to become part of the workings of another system may provide, as Bowers proposes, the direction to be taken in formulating a new paradigm to replace the one according to which so many of the new research findings are inexplicable if not anomalous.

Rossi outlines how many of the major pathways of brain activity involved with memory, learning, and behavior support the view that the limbic-hypothalamus system is the primary mind/body transducer. After introducing the concept of state-dependent learning and memory—that what is learned and remembered is "dependent on one's psychosociological state at the time of the experience" (Rossi [1986] 1993:47)—he explores evidence supporting the transduction and flow of information to and from the psyche and other systems, such as the autonomic nervous, endocrine, immune, and neuropeptide systems.

Elsewhere, Rossi cites an experimental study by Glaser et al. (1993, 1990) demonstrating the negative effect of stress experienced by medical students during academic examinations on their immune systems by tracing its effect on the transcription of the interleukin-2 receptor gene. By measuring how "information transduction is modulated by psychological stress throughout the main cellular-genetic loop of information transduction," Glaser and his associates, according to Rossi (Rossi and Rossi 1996:102), were able to demonstrate how psychosocial processes of mind and behavior can be related to genetic expression.

Independent confirmation came from a number of studies in the new field of psychoneuroimmunology, a term coined by Robert Ader, an experimental psychologist. Ader and his colleague Nicholas Cohen (Ader and Cohen 1991) showed "that the immune system can be trained, *or conditioned*, to respond to a neutral stimulus" (Rodgers 2006:284; emphasis in original). Medication and placebos were tried; it was shown that patients responded positively when told that what they were being given (or what was being done to them) would make them better.

Rossi drew on a study conducted on an island in Venezuela in which children suffering from asthma were divided into two groups, one given relaxation and guided imagery exercises, plus therapy to improve their self-esteem, and the other given nothing. The "number of asthmatic episodes and the use of bronchodilator medication used in the group exposed to the psychosocial intervention were significantly reduced, and pulmonary function was significantly improved" (Castés et al. 1999:1). There was also a significant reduction in the specific molecular responses against the most important allergen in these children. None of these changes were seen in the other group.

Later studies of laboratory animals led to the questioning of this simple relationship between stress and depressed immune function in humans (Dantzer 1997; Dhabhar et al. 1995). They led to the conclusion that acute stress can be separated from chronic stress, which is usually associated with depression. The former, it appears, redistributes peripheral blood leukocytes (in rats) to other bodily compartments, serving to enhance immune surveillance and ultimately immune function (Dabhar and McEwen 1996:2608). Only chronic stress, the kind with which Rossi is concerned, depresses immune function.

The basic assumption of this argument for the influence of the psychosocial on the biological, supported by much ongoing research, is the opposite of that found in so much of the current literature written by students of contemporary genetics. Contrary to the ontological priority that has been attributed to the genes by the new molecular biology since Francis Crick first formulated the "central dogma" of DNA $\longrightarrow$ RNA $\longrightarrow$ protein (Lewontin et al. 1984:58; see also Crick 1958)—which, based on the old mechanical imagery, supports genetic reductionism—the position taken here is that it is the combination of information from genes, but also from sources external to genes, even external to the organism, that accounts for most of the organism's behavior. In terms of the new information/communication imagery, nature and nurture are taken to be ontologically coterminous. When we focus on interrelatedness and communication between parts, neither alone fully determines what the organism does.

Unfortunately, the nature/nurture debate, since its beginnings, has been formulated in terms of the Cartesian dualism and the assumption that if treated at all, res cognitas phenomena must be reduced to res extensa. As in the formulation of science being challenged, the material that was studied scientifically and known, in this case the biological, was opposed to a catchall external category labeled "environment." From the perspective of biology, and the medicine based on it, including early psychology, this nonspecific category is opposed to a specific entity (or property) whose importance and influence is theorized in the search for a reductionist explanatory theory. This in part led Black, Bowers, Pert, Rossi, and others attempting to reformulate the mind/body dualism in terms of a nonmechanical, communication/information metaphor not to recognize, let alone include, the importance of ,and role played by, humanity's self-created environment: culture.

In the development of medicine, a black box was placed over mind, leading to medicine's emphasis on the soma and biology. When it was removed, mind was taken to mean the brain and became the province of psychology. Generally, the fields of sociology and anthropology did not participate in the mind/body debate or in the effort to reconceptualize the dualism. Medical anthropology was the exception, but even it has not directly confronted the challenge. Moreover, the influence of psychiatry led its practitioners to give priority to the individual as they attempted to add an understanding of culture to the practice of medicine.

At the end of chapter 6, I questioned whether standard anthropological analyses of ritual healing could explain Kardecist surgeries and disobsessions, since patient and healer did not necessarily share a cosmology, values, contexts, and systems of semiosis at the time of treatment. The same question could be asked about the ritual healings of the other religions discussed in part II. Many of those treated who report success and convert learn the specific beliefs of the group only during the healing ritual. How can they embody aspects of a worldview claimed to precipitate a transformation in them when they do not already share the belief system? More importantly, if we follow Rossi's framework, how is the information presented in the ritual transduced to affect the body and make it well?

To answer these questions, I turn to anthropology's traditional view of culture, treating its content as information. In this way, I will be able to build on what Rossi and the others have already accomplished and offer an expanded imagery for the new paradigm. I call it culturalbiology.

Culture is the term anthropologists use to refer to all those aspects of human cognition and behavior that cannot be accounted for by the information and instructions contained in the genetic materials transferred from parent to offspring in the reproductive process. When, in the late nineteenth century, he set out what was to become an academic discipline, Sir Edward B. Tylor defined what has become its master concept as "that complex whole which includes knowledge, belief, art, morals, law, custom, and any other capabilities and habits *acquired by man as a member of society*" ([1871] 1958(1):1; italics added) Later, A. L. Kroeber would add: "Anthropology is the interrelation of what is biological in man and what is social and historical in him" ([1921] 1948:2). From its beginnings, anthropology has been a field straddling the sciences and the humanities and concerned with the relative interdependence and balance between the biological and the cultural in human behavior.

Early field studies revealed the broad range of diversity in the organization of human lives, leading anthropologists to emphasize the differences between peoples and raising questions about the cultural and behavioral potential that biology made possible. Prior to World War II, as Wolf observes, "the psychobiological design of man seemed irrelevant" (1974:33). It was assumed to be open and "could be made to subscribe to any culture. Cultural variability, unhampered by limitations of physique or psyche, seemed endless." Emphasis was placed on the range of socially based cultural learning acquired by an individual as a member of society, almost to the neglect of possible biological limitations. This orientation changed significantly after the Second World War.

Humans came to be seen as forced by the inherited design "over and over again to seek answers to the same questions, solutions to the same needs" (Wolf 1974:33). This postwar change as to how much genetic underpinnings determined or constrained human potential to create culture coincided with the genetic revolution. Students focusing exclusively on the body in the Cartesian dualism formed new fields such as sociobiology and evolutionary psychology and berated anthropology, claiming that it paid no attention to the biological design of the human animal. Using older anthropological studies and discussions of learned behavior as "straw men," they continue to criticize the field in their effort to reduce explanations of human behavior to biology.

This assault was and continues to be unnecessary. Recent theory and research in neuroscience emphatically shows that "*nature and nurture are always interacting in the processes of psychobiological communication via the psychosocial dynamics of gene expression*" (Rossi 2002:201; emphasis in original). Neuroscience would profit by adding the culturalbiological imagery and the comparative cultural perspective that anthropology has brought to scientific inquiry, while anthropology would benefit from the addition of more biophysiology when planning research and analyzing data.

In a series of papers attempting to integrate psychiatry with developments in brain studies and genetics, Nobel laureate neuropsychologist Eric Kandel (1999, 1998) expresses the nonreductionist perspective of contemporary anthropology in his discussion of gene expression:

> The regulation of gene expression by social factors makes all bodily functions, including all functions of the brain, susceptible to social influences. These social influences will be biologically incorporated in the altered expressions of specific genes in specific nerve cells of specific regions of the brain. These socially influenced alterations are transmitted culturally. They are not incorporated in the sperm and egg and therefore are not transmitted genetically. In humans the modifiability of gene expression through learning (in a non-transmissible way) is particularly effective and has led to a new kind of evolution: cultural evolution. (Kandel 1998:461)

Kandel observes further that "the capability of learning is so highly developed in humans that humankind changes much more by cultural evolution than by biological evolution" (1998:461). Moreover, the content of learned culture varies across social groups that share most of their genetic materials.

The major characteristic of humans is their capacity to symbolize. Symbols are a class of signs whose relationship to their referents—what they stand for and the meanings given them—is arbitrary and determined by those who use them. Each social group over time has developed its own symbolic categories, patterns of normative cultural conduct, and the symbolic means for representing and understanding them.

Since elders do not always intentionally and/or consciously transmit to each new generation the rules for cultural performance and the resultant complex of appropriate behaviors, we may ask: How does it happen? What are the mechanisms by which the symbolic information that is culture is passed on to, and interacts with, the genetically transmitted biophysiological instructions that result in socially applicable but individually diverse behavior? Two developments help clarify the answer. The first relates to information flow and the ability of the human organism to absorb it. The second concerns a major class of genes, sometimes called immediate-early or primary response genes, that are the specific mediators between learned behavior from the psychocultural domain and all other genes.

"*What we perceive at any moment,*" writes Manfred Zimmermann,[42] "*is limited to an extremely small compartment in the stream of information about our surroundings flowing in from the sense organs*" (Nørretranders 1998:124, quoting Zimmermann1989; emphasis in Nørretranders). Elsewhere, Zimmermann elaborates:

> The maximal information flow of the process of conscious sensory perception is about 40 bits/[second]—many orders of magnitude below that taken in by receptors [nerve endings]. Our perception, then, would appear to be limited to a minute part of the abundance of information available as sensory input. (Zimmermann 1986:116)

Millions of bits of information flood through the human senses every single second. Zimmermann estimates some 10 million bits per second entering through the eyes, another million through the skin, 100,000 each through the ears and nose, and still another thousand through the taste buds (1989:172). Of this more than 11 million bits of information per second, human beings appear to be consciously aware of, at most, approximately 40 bits. The remainder either is discarded—lost for practical purposes—or organized (in terms of the categories of the specific culture), and then either used or stored for later retrieval without conscious (and reflexive) awareness.

With respect to immediate-early genes, Trölle et al. write:

> Recent advances in cellular biology have identified the activation and deactivation of immediate-early genes as molecular mechanisms to control regulated and deregulated growth, cellular differentiation and development. In this view immediate-early genes may function as third messengers in a stimulus transcription cascade transferring extracellular information into changes in target gene transcription, thereby changing the phenotype of neurons. (Trölle et al. 1995:preface)

Or, as Rossi notes, immediate-early genes

> are actively turned on and off every second of our lives in response to the hormonal messenger molecules that carry information that is important for the continual process of adaptation to our current

environment. Everything from sexual stimuli, temperature, food, psychological stress, physical trauma and toxins in the environment can be signaled to the genes. (Rossi 1998:2; see also Merchant 1996)

Rossi continues elsewhere:

Most arousing environmental stimuli that have been studied can induce immediate-early genes within minutes, their concentrations typically peak within fifteen to twenty minutes and their effects usually over within an hour or two. The changes in gene transcription and new protein formation initiated in this time frame, however, can lead to lasting changes in the central nervous system by converting short-term memory to lasting learning. (Rossi 1998:3, citing Bailey, Bartsch, and Kandel 1996; Tully 1996)

This unspecified environment of the individual whose genes are being turned on and off includes the culture of his or her group. Some of the information embedded in its cultural codes, which provide meaning and understanding to members of a community or society, is transduced, most often without the conscious (reflexive) awareness of the individual, to become part of the information flow that influences the physical body and its constituent systems by activating immediate-early genes.

Before proceeding, it would be useful to introduce the distinction made by neurobiologists between conscious or declarative learning and memory, on the one hand, and procedural or implicit (nondeclarative) learning and memory, as used by psychologists and psychoanalysts (LeDoux 2002:chs. 5, 6; Milner, Squire, and Kandel 1998). Declarative learning and memory are conscious and usually easy for an individual to recall and present verbally. Declarative learning refers to people, objects, and places. Nondeclarative or implicit memory and learning are the ways we act and our perceptual and motor skills. They are not conscious, often difficult if not impossible to express verbally, and evident only in performance rather than in recall (LeDoux 2002:98; Kandel 1999:508). Through repetition, declarative memory can be transformed into the procedural type. An example is learning to drive a car, which at first involves conscious recollection but eventually becomes an automatic and nonconscious motor activity (Kandel 1999:508). Cognitive anthropologist Roy D'Andrade's opposition between connectionist and serial logic parallels this distinction between conscious and procedural learning and memory (D'Andrade

1995; see also Strauss and Quinn 1994; Bloch 1991).

D'Andrade places both forms of logic within a schema that he defines as "the organization of cognitive elements into abstract mental objects capable of being held in working memory with default values or open slots which can be variously filled with appropriate specifics" (D'Andrade 1995:179). Serial or sentential logic recodes experience into symbols, while parallel connectionist logic transforms it in connections between neuronlike units (D'Andrade, 1995:140). The two forms of logic lead to two ways of learning, with serial logic being more explicit and much quicker, since it can be verbalized in terms of rules. The connectionist logic leads to a more permanent result and more rapid and automatic execution (D'Andrade 1995:144).

Many aspects of culture learned early in life, such as music and language, are learned implicitly. Consequently, rarely are they ever brought to the level of consciousness. Examples abound. It is well documented that when people from sub-Saharan Africa walk or dance, their hips and lower limbs alone seem to be in motion. Europeans, in contrast, employ their heads, shoulders, and legs. One pattern has no adaptive advantage over the other, since both enable the individual to go from one place to another or to rhythmically accompany music. This fact does not stop members of either group from ridiculing those among them who do not act "properly." That is, members of social groups judge and then sanction each other when one does not conform to patterns that are normative to the group. The behaviors, as in the case of language, are learned in emotion-laden contexts, making them, in Rossi's sense, state dependent.

This is true of other seemingly mundane aspects of life, such as eating or covering the body. Certainly, at a basic biological level, humans are capable of consuming and deriving nutrition from a wide variety of items. In fact, specific societies consume only a limited range of things available to them. Furthermore, their members often respond negatively to even the thought of ingesting, let alone swallowing, what they have been taught is not food. Conversely, many foods are associated with strong positive feelings. In instances where populations have been incorporated as minorities in modern nations, foods they believe to have been eaten regularly by their ancestors have on occasions become markers of (ethnic) identity. The emotionality associated with their consumption suggests that learning to ingest them may have been state dependent.

We may claim that biological processes make us "feel hungry" at appropriate times. When a meal is missed because of pressing activities or travel in parts of the world where three meals a day are not standard, we become hungry according to our schedule and react when deprived of access to food. A similar response frequently occurs when fully nutritious exotic foods are offered. Even if we are very hungry, accepting insects or rats as food could result in uncontrollable biological reactions.

A great variety of distinctively human behaviors, including how people think about the world in which they live and the categories they use to classify what is in it—"the belief[s], art, morals, law, custom, and . . . other capabilities and habits acquired by man as a member of society," set out by Tylor [1871] (1958:1:1) to define culture—are learned implicitly and encoded in a state-dependent manner. Although not necessarily available to consciousness or for discussion, they are present, ordering the thinking and activities of those exposed to (or socialized in terms of) the learning patterns of a particular group. Held in the declarative memories of individual members of a group, they appear more in shared symbols and images than in words.

Cultures, as shown previously for Klass's East Indian peasants and the Brazilian Kardecists, popular Catholics, Candombléiros, Umbandistas, and Pentecostals, contain views of the cosmos that include understandings as to what exists and what has causal efficacy with respect to the life of the individual. Sacred symbols, writes Geertz,

> function to synthesize a people's ethos—the tone, character, and quality of their life, its moral and aesthetic style and mood—and their world view—the picture they have of the way things in sheer actuality are, their most comprehensive ideas of order. In religious belief and practice a group's ethos is rendered intellectually reasonable by being shown to represent a way of life ideally adapted to the actual state of affairs the world view describes, while the world view is rendered emotionally convincing by being presented as an image of an actual state of affairs peculiarly well-arranged to accommodate such a way of life. ...
>
> ...The notion that religion tunes human actions to an envisaged cosmic order and projects images of cosmic order onto the plane of human experience is hardy novel. But it is hardly investigated

either, so that we have very little idea of how, in empirical terms this particular miracle is accomplished. (Geertz 1973:89–90)

These beliefs are more than superstition. By focusing on the information they contain and how it may be transduced, via the brain of someone who accepts them, to other bodily systems—to the level of the cell and genes—we may discover that cultural beliefs are part of the communication system that instructs the T cells and killer cells of the immune system, for example, to attack the pathogens that cause somatic illness. Franz Ingelfinger, former editor of the *New England Journal of Medicine*, informs us that "85 percent of all the illnesses physicians are called upon to treat are self-limiting. That is, without any help, the human body is able in most cases to prescribe for itself" (Cousins 1986:ix).

Religious rituals, as Lévi-Strauss (1966, 1963), Turner ([1964] 1979, 1969, 1967), and others have emphasized, are forms of communication, perhaps, as Goodman (1988:33) observes, "the most exalted form of human communication." In the course of their unfolding, information about what she calls the "other reality," with its powerful forces and beings, is communicated to the participants. Rituals, as psychologist Stanley Krippner notes, "are ways in which mythological themes are performed" (2005:97). They embody "storehouses of meaningful symbols by which information is revealed and regarded as authoritative." (Turner 1968:2). This stating "of sacra," as Turner adds elsewhere in his discussion of ritual initiation,

> both teaches the neophytes how to think with some degree of abstraction about their cultural milieu [and the forces in it] and gives them ultimate standards of reference. At the same time, it is believed to change their nature, transform them from one kind of a human being into another. (Turner [1964] 1979:242)

Traditional (shamanic and other) rituals and practices, add Frecska and Kulcsar, have as their end the destruction of what they refer to as profane sensibilities:

> The monotonous chants, the endless repeated refrains, the fatigue, the fasting, the dancing . . . create a sensory condition that is wide open to the "supernatural." This is not only . . . a matter of physiological techniques: traditional ideology directs and imparts values to all these efforts intended to break the frame of profane sensibility.

> What is above all indispensable is the absolute belief of the sub-
> ject in the spiritual universe that he desires to enter. (Frecska and
> Kulcsar 1989:70; see also Eliade 1976:85)

Outlining the universal structure of what Moerman (1979) called
symbolic healing, Dow proposes a series of stages through which
healing rituals pass:

> (1) A generalized cultural mythic world is established by universal-
> izing the experiences of healers, initiates, or prophets, or by otherwise
> generalizing emotional experiences. (2) A healer persuades the patient
> that it is possible to define the patient's relationship to a particularized
> part of the mythic world, and makes the definition. (3) The healer
> attaches the patient's emotions to transactional symbols in this par-
> ticularized mythic world. (4) The healer manipulates the transactional
> symbols to assist the transaction of emotion. (Dow 1986:66)

The substance or content (conceptualized here as information) of
a group's shared understandings as to what exists and has efficacy in
the universe—contained in the belief system of its culture—may be
thought of as first learned and then carried in the implicit or nondeclarative memories of the individual members of the group. Each
person would not necessarily be consciously aware of it,[43] and there
would be no need for it to be accessed verbally in the ordinary waking state. But it is there, often in imagery, and, as Aijmer elaborates,
may have some dramatic implications:

> People in interaction always draw on their repository of images
> when they construct social life. The force of imagery is something
> which is not easily retrievable in terms of language. ... Images
> make themselves known through cultural institutions, not by way
> of reflexive thought.
> ... Imagery, especially in the form of stable icons, frames and
> supports the social discourse. The force it transmits being differ-
> ently construed than the sentences of language, gives a particular
> dignity—the voice of human morality—to its messages, which are
> clearly intuited and yet not reflexively understood. ...
> It seems to operate mentally more like visual pictures than for-
> mulations in words, and its semanticity hinges on the simultaneous
> presence of elements that are in themselves images. ... If an actor
> constructs a great part of his scenarios as a resultant of his social
> review, he also calls on his social cognizance (for want of a better

term) of cultural imagery, thereby drawing into his acts implications of morality, righteousness, correctness, order, and ultimately the force of blessing. (Aijmer 1995:4–5)

Stoller's studies on the role of music and dance in conveying information, and their meaning in healing rituals among the Songhay, add further support to the argument (Stoller 1996; see also Basso 1985).

I propose that information stored in the implicit memory of members of a society, of which the individual is not necessarily consciously aware, then can be transduced via the brain into the codes of bodily systems to trigger the rest of what Rossi ([1986] 1993:140–60) presents in his model of brain/body communication.[44]

We now have a mechanism by which the transformative model of medical anthropology works, articulating ritual and its content with biophysiology. When a suffering individual is treated during a healing ritual, the cultural images in the universe believed to be able to heal him or her, often conceptualized as spirits and other supernatural beings, are brought forth from the person's implicit memory and, as information, transduced, first into psychological codes and then into biophysiological codes, and communicated through the body. This information turns on immediate-early genes that produce proteins and other chemicals to communicate with and activate the immune, neuropeptide, and other systems that inhibit pain, fight infections, or do whatever else might contribute to the abatement of symptoms. By adding the role of culture and its mostly nonverbalized but implicitly held, powerful other reality learned by members as part of religious rituals (Goodman 1988:33) to Rossi's model, we may finally have, to use his words, "the common denominator between traditional Western medicine and the holistic, shamanistic, and spiritualistic approaches to healing that depend upon highly specialized cultural belief systems, world views, and frames of reference" (Rossi [1986] 1993:68).

CHAPTER 17

RITUAL, ALTERED STATES OF CONSCIOUSNESS, AND IMPLEMENTING CULTURALBIOLOGICAL HEALING

Hypnosis, a word derived from the Greek *hypnos*, meaning "sleep," was a central feature of healing at early Greek temples. It came into modern medicine in the work of Franz Anton Mesmer a little over two centuries ago. This was just before the advent of chemical anesthesia, modern psychology, psychiatry, and psychoanalysis. After being adopted by French colleagues Charcot, Janet, Bernheim, and others, "magnetic healing" was brought to England, where Scotsman James Braid reformulated it and renamed it hypnosis (Inglis 1989:61). After a period of discontinuance in its use and study, Hull, Erickson, and Hilgard in the United States revived research, while Milton Erickson reintroduced its application in therapy (Gauld 1992).

A central feature of hypnotically facilitated healing is that the therapist makes a series of suggestions to a patient that are intended to induce physical and/or emotional changes that will ameliorate specific symptoms. In contrast with other treatment forms, in hypnotherapy the patient is believed to be in a state (of mind) different from normal.

In the 1950s, Arthur Mason applied hypnosis to effectively treat a sixteen-year-old with warts. "Within 10 days the wart fell off and normal skin replaced it" (Rodgers 2006, citing Mason and Black 1958).

In the 1980s T. X. Barber (1984) summarized a series of studies that showed changes in (assumedly unchangeable) bodily processes in response to hypnotic interventions, which resulted in a reduction in, or elimination of, a number of illnesses. Barber (1984:106) concluded that

> believed-in suggestions, which are incorporated into ongoing suggestions, affect blood supply in localized areas, and the altered blood flow, in turn, plays a role in producing some of the phenomena ...described. ... Specifically, the altered blood flow may play an important role in 1) reducing the dermatitis produced by a poison ivy-like plant, 2) giving rise to a degree of dermatitis when the poisonous plant is not actually present, 3) producing localized skin inflammation that has the specific pattern of a previously experienced burn, 4) curing warts that have been present for a long period of time, 5) ameliorating congenital ichthyosis, 6) stimulating the enlargement of the mammary gland, 7) producing bruises by suggestions, 8) minimizing bleeding after exodontia, etc., and 9) minimizing and also enlarging the effects of a burn. (Barber 1984:106)

A decade later, Holroyd, citing additional studies that reported the ability of hypnotized individuals to control bleeding, modify blood flow to various parts of the body, activate immune response, control pain, and affect the central nervous system, contributing to healing, agreed that "hypnosis and suggestion have demonstrated remarkable clinical effects" (Holroyd 1992:207).[45]

In the practice of medicine, hypnotically facilitated therapy has been used as anesthesia or to alter the flow of blood going to a specific part of the body in order to ameliorate a particular condition (Barber

1984; Ewin 1984; Moore and Kaplan 1983; Marmer 1959). It has been reported to lower stressors such as adrenaline, noradrenaline, and cortisone and to stimulate the body's own painkillers, the beta-endorphins (Goodman 1988:39), and the immune system (Ruzyla-Smith et al. 1995; Ley and Freeman 1984). It has been found to help patients suffering from irritable bowel syndrome (Gonsalkorale et al. 2003; Gonsalkorale, Houghton, and Whorwell 2002) and to improve the quality of life of those suffering from anxiety and depression (Gonsalkorale, Toner, and Whorwell 2004).

Anthropologists have examined similar phenomena, calling them trance and spirit possession in small-scale societies or religious groups. Erika Bourguinon (1976) differentiated between "possession," "possession trance," and "trance." She wrote that possession occurs when a spirit produces alterations in someone's behavior, health, or disposition without changes in awareness. Possession trance happens if the host loses consciousness and demonstrates the behavior, speech patterns, and body movements of the spirit said to inhabit it. Trance is an altered state of consciousness in which a person does not have an awareness of an outside agent inhabiting or taking over his or her body. Although interesting and important for other problems, I find these distinctions, and the literature that builds on them, of little help in answering the questions posed in this book and explaining the anomalous therapies used by the religious groups in Brazil.

Unfortunately, the conscious awareness and intent of the person exhibiting the special state has been the focus of much of the debate about hypnosis. Barber (Chaves and Barber 1974), for example, who originally maintained that the effect was obtained by little more than the "hypnotist" making suggestions in a situation where the party acted on was strongly motivated to do what the other requested, more recently has set out three categories or types of people he calls good hypnotic subjects: 1) individuals who are fantasy prone; 2) those who are amnesia prone and forget memorable events in their lives; and 3) people defined as "positively-set . . . with strongly positive attitudes, motivations, expectancies, and cognitions toward the hypnotic test situation" (Barber 1999).

Hypnotic induction, according to most researchers, turns on a special relationship established between two parties, one who is being hypnotized and another who performs the induction and makes the suggestions. The subject, or patient in the context of therapy, must respect authority generally and that of his dyadic partner in the hypnotic setting.

In Brazil, the culture, across variability in ethnic traditions, social classes, religious groups, and other localized manifestations, teaches, emphasizes, reinforces, and rewards fantasy:

> Children (and adults) who claim to see the Virgin Mary, Saint Francis, some other saint, or other supernatural beings not only are not punished or taken to a therapist ... but are rewarded and held up for praise. Those who claim to "receive" a spirit, whether a doctor from the past like Adolph Fritz ... or a deity from Africa such as Iemanja, Oxala, etc. in Candomble, Xango or Batuque, or the spirit of a former slave (a preto velho) or an Indian (a caboclo) as in Umbanda . . . not only are believed, but their help is sought by others who treat them deferentially and with respect. (Greenfield 1991:23)

Moreover, the culture's traditional pattern of structuring interpersonal relations in terms of hierarchically ordered patron–client ties (see Roniger 1990, 1987; Greenfield 1979a, 1977b, 1972; Hutchinson 1966), which have been carried over into all the religious practices examined in parts 1 and 2 (Greenfield and Cavalcante 2006), results in something similar to the ideal relationship between hypnotist and client/subject, but perhaps stronger because the ties are institutionalized and do not have to be established anew in each hypnotic encounter. Those participating in religious rituals in the hope of being helped are highly motivated and fantasy prone and stand in the structural relationship of dependency vis-à-vis a trusted authority offering healing and help.

Brazilian psychotherapist David Akstein, a specialist in hypnosis and hypnotherapy, recognized the role of trance or altered states in the healing practices of Brazilian popular religions almost three decades ago when he wrote about "terpsichoretrance" as a form of therapy (Akstein 1977, 1973). He maintains that during public rituals such as carnival, and more importantly when participating in the sessions of spiritualist sects, individuals enter into trance states. He calls those that happen during religious rituals—as opposed to carnival—kinetic trances. In this state, he contends, "certain patients develop sudden and diffuse inhibition of the cerebral cortex, generating reciprocal induction of the emotional centers" (Akstein 1977:222; see also Akstein 1973, 1965). That is, in religiously induced trance, a level of cerebral cortex inhibition that facilitates suggestibility is obtained. The altered states, he maintains, have a deep and intense "therapeutic effect on the followers" (Akstein 1977:221).

Unlike Akstein, with his interest in his native Brazilian popular religions, most researchers who study hypnosis and hypnotic states belong to a culture that assumes a world of autonomous individuals, each in control of his or her own actions.[46] Behavior over which the individual appears not to have control, or that differs from his or her "ordinary" behavior, often is said to be the result of the person being in an altered state of consciousness (ASC). "The traditions of European peoples and their New World descendants," as Winkelman (2000:3) reminds us, "have tended to deprecate ASC in their emphasis on rational thought." Some of its advocates even contend that hypnosis is an ASC (Matthews, Lankton, and Lankton 1993:190; Bowers 1966; Hilgard 1966; Gill and Brenman 1959; Orne 1959). When it is applied in therapy, the party being treated is induced into such a state. The therapist gives suggestions containing information that may be transduced to activate the endocrine or immune system, reduce stress, or alter the flow of blood, all contributing to the patient's cure.

The assumption that there are ASCs presupposes the existence of a regular or customary mode. Western scientists refer to this mode as the normal waking state, during which the individual acts "rationally" and is in control. A consequence of this assumption is that those who do not behave as expected by others with whom they interact or who study them are said to be in an ASC. As Goodman reminds us, people who enter such states, for example during the performance of religious rituals, until recently "had the dubious distinction of being …singled out by Western psychiatry as being abnormal and hence insane" (Goodman 1988:36).[47]

Anthropologists generally have accepted this formulation of a normal state versus alternate ones. Consequently, they write about the people they study, especially those interacting with supernatural beings while participating in religious rituals, as being in an ASC.

Bourguignon and her students demonstrated many years ago that

most human beings enter into altered states regularly in the performance of religious rituals. In a sample of 488 small-scale societies,
she found that almost 90 percent showed evidence of religious trance
behavior (Bourguignon and Evascu 1977; Bourguignon 1973, 1968).
"Unless one wanted to maintain that the overwhelming majority of
humanity was insane . . . the conclusion," according to one of her students, "was inescapable that religious trance was a perfectly normal
human experience" (Goodman 1988:36). Goodman continues:

> We need to add an important qualifier here, however. *Institutional-*
> *ized* religious trances are normal. That is, when and if the trance
> represents controlled behavior, when it is *ritualized action*, capable
> of being called forth and terminated on a given cue or signal, *then*
> it is a perfectly normal phenomenon. (Goodman 1988:36; emphasis
> in the original)[48]

While some still question whether a state such as hypnosis—and
by implication all altered states—actually exists and contend that if
it does, only a small percentage of people are "good" hypnotic subjects and able to respond with or without formal induction, (Rossi
2002, [1986] 1993; E. Rossi and K. Rossi 1996), following in the
tradition of Erickson, maintains that entering an altered state is part
of the normal, everyday, biological experience of all human beings.
Rossi (E. Rossi and K. Rossi 1996:120) refers to this situation as
"the wave nature of consciousness and being." He notes that half a
century ago, researchers observed that every ninety minutes or so
throughout the night, sleep became a very "active process" for about
ten to thirty minutes, during which oxygen consumption increased
and more blood flowed to the brain. Breathing, heart rate, blood
pressure, and gastrointestinal movements became more variable than
during wakefulness. During these periods of rapid eye movement
(REM), sleep brain wave patterns, as measured by electroencephalo-
graph (EEG), became similar to active waking patterns. Researchers
later confirmed that the 90- to 120-minute dream rhythm apparently continues during the day. Kleitman (1982, 1969, 1963), one of
the first to observe the REM activity pattern, refers to a basic rest-
activity cycle (BRAC) in sleep and wakefulness.

The early therapists using hypnosis, according to Rossi (Rossi and
Rossi 1996:124) were intuitively aware of the wave nature of human

experience. But it was Milton Erickson who effectively applied it. Unlike his colleagues who saw patients for a fifty-minute session, Erickson preferred to meet for an hour and a half or more. "He claimed that people in everyday life also naturally drifted between subtle but distinct mindbody states. When he worked with patients for at least an hour and a half or two, he found, they were almost certain to go through distinct changes in their consciousness and states of being" (Rossi and Rossi 1996:129):

> During these lengthier sessions, for no apparent reason, the patient's head might start to nod rhythmically; eyelids would blink slowly, and then close over faraway-looking eyes. The body might go perfectly still, with fingers, hands, or legs apparently frozen in an awkward position. Sometimes there was a subtle smile on the person's face or, more often, the features were passive and slack. ... On some occasions, Erickson did nothing to direct people to go into trance; it just seemed to happen, sooner or later, all by itself. (Rossi and Rossi 1996:129)

Erickson called these natural periods the common everyday trance. They are times of "openness and vulnerability to outside influences; suggestions made during this time are sometimes more easily accepted" (Rossi and Rossi 1996:130).

Figure 1 illustrates Rossi's hypothesis that "the natural unit of psychobiologically oriented psychotherapy is the utilization of one of the 90–120 minute cycles of activity and rest" illustrated in the lower part of the figure (Rossi 2002:69; see also Rossi and Rossi 1996, Lloyd and Rossi 1992). This 90 to 120 minutes is the time it takes for the gene expression/protein synthesis cycle to complete one ultradian cycle of healing on the level of "psychosocial genomics," which he hypothesizes is the molecular basis of mind/body healing. Based on it, Rossi affirms that,

> *what has been traditionally called "therapeutic suggestion" may be, in essence, the accessing, entrainment, and utilization of ultradian/circadian replays of mind-body communication on all levels, from the cellular-genomic to the behavioral, that are responsive to psychosocial cues.* (Rossi 2002:70; italics in the original)

Figure 1. The Four-Stage Creative Process in
Psychobiologically Oriented Psychotherapy

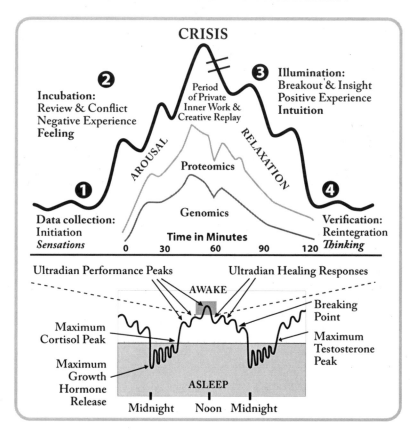

From Rossi (2002:68):

The lower diagram summarizes the alternating 90–120 minute ultradian rhythms of waking and sleeping for an entire day in a simplified manner. The ascending peaks of rapid eye movement (REM) sleep characteristic of nightly dreams every 90–120 minutes or so are illustrated along with the more variable ultradian rhythms of activity, adaptation, and rest in the daytime. This lower figure also illustrates how many hormonal messenger molecules of the endocrine system, such as *growth hormone,* the activating and stress hormone cortisol, and the sexual hormone testosterone, have typical circadian peaks at different times of the 24-hour cycle.

The upper diagram outlines the basic psychobiological unit of psychotherapy as the creative utilization of one of the natural 90–120 minute ultradian rhythms of arousal and relaxation illustrated in the lower diagram.

In *The Psychobiology of Mind-Body Healing* ([1986] 1993), Rossi proposed that hypnotherapy (or hypnotically facilitated therapy) may activate bodily systems at the cellular and even genetic levels that can contribute to the healing of a variety of illnesses traditionally categorized as physical, as well as those labeled psychosomatic. He begins his argument by presenting evidence to demonstrate that the placebo is still perhaps the most successful long-term treatment modality in medicine.[49] He contends that when an individual believes something will help him or her, that knowledge, as information, may be transduced to activate other bodily systems, down to the level of the cells and genes, analogous to the way pharmaceuticals work. One of Rossi's primary objectives is to show how hypnotherapy can contribute to healing both when complementing conventional treatments and on its own. He adds,

> It is the *patient's own internal hypnotherapeutic work* rather than the therapist's hypnotic suggestions or programming per se that is the essence of hypnosis in problem solving and healing. (Rossi and Rossi 1996:119; italics in the original)[50]

Anthropologist Michael Winkelman, writing about ASC from a comparative, cross-cultural perspective, adds:

> The common psychophysiological changes of ASC—parasympathetic dominance, inter-hemispheric integration, and limbic-frontal synchronization—can be seen as having therapeutic effects *sui generis*. The parasympathetic dominant state synchronization of the frontal cortex, and inter-hemispheric integration area associated with conditions of psychophysiological integration and coordination (limbic-frontal and left-right hemisphere) have inherent benefits for the functioning of the human system. The parasympathetic-dominant state reflects a basic relaxation response characterized by an integrated hypothalamic response and a generalized decrease in the activation of the sympathetic nervous system. This is the basic lack of response to counteract the overactivity of the sympathetic

nervous system. The relaxation response has preventive and thera-peutic value in diseases characterized by increased sympathetic ner-vous system activity. (Winkelman 1997:405)

Based on this and Rossi's work, the model of culturalbiology pre-sented in chapter 16 hypothesizes that healing and other benefits to a suffering individual occur when information at the cultural level, held as beliefs (that interrupt habitual patterns of association) as to what in the universe has the ability to cause and cure illness or resolve other problems, such as spirits, saints, orixás, and the Holy Ghost (in their specific cosmological settings), is transduced via the psyche of a participant in a religious ritual. The beliefs of (traditional) non-Western peoples and some religious groups, like those discussed in this volume, as to what has power both to cause illness and to cure it, viewed as information held at the implicit level, are comparable to what practitioners of hypnotically facilitated therapy explicitly pres-ent to their (Western) patients as suggestions. When, in controlled situations, members of these religious or traditional groups enter into what Goodman (1988) calls religious ASC and continue uninter-rupted for at least one 90 to 120 minute cycle of activity and rest (BRAC), they may be undergoing the same process of psychosocial genomics as hypnotized patients. In terms of Rossi's model, they may transduce sufficient information into their bodily systems to (1) turn on immediate-early genes that, as shown in figure 2, "(2) may lead to the expression of specific target genes, which (3) code for new protein synthesis that is the molecular basis of (4) state-dependent memory, learning, behavior (SDMLB) that is replayed on conscious and unconscious levels" (Rossi 2002:200).

We have seen that considerable evidence exists to support the idea of the transduction of information from the symbolic level to physi-ological processes in healing when hypnosis is applied in medical practice (see also Brown 1992; Brown and Fromm 1987). In hypnoti-cally facilitated therapy, the precipitating information is passed from one party, the therapist, in the form of suggestions, to a second party, who accepts or believes what the other party is saying. In treatment by shamans and other so-called traditional healers, such as the Kardecist mediums, pais- and mães-de-santo in Candomblé and Umbanda, and Pentecostal pastors, suggestions are not necessarily made explicitly to an individual. Instead, information, such as the belief that a spirit, an orixá, a preto velho, or the Holy Spirit will help a sufferer with his problem, often presented in testimonials given by those already helped, is made known explicitly to all present. When a suffering participant's own ultradian, 90 to 120 minute gene expression/protein synthesis cycle falls within the time frame of the ritual, could it be that the information presented and/or brought forth into active memory is transduced to join the information flow of the participant's body, turning on immediate-early genes, directing the flow of blood, and activating the immune and other biological systems that relieve pain and lead to healing?[51] Could this be the explanation for the otherwise inexplicable surgeries and other healings?

FIGURE 2. A PSYCHOGENOMIC VIEW OF
THE PSYCHOSOMATIC NETWORK

Psychobiological Arousal

Pain, Stress, Novelty, BRAC,
REM Sleep, Creative Moments,
and the Numinosum

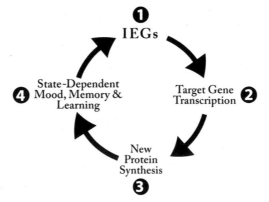

From Rossi (2002:200):

Mindbody communication via the dynamics of psychobiological arousal that can initiate (1) immediate early gene expression (IEG) that, in turn, leads to (2) the expression of specific target genes, which (3) code for new protein synthesis that is the molecular basis of (40 state-dependent memory, learning, behavior (SDMLB) that is replayed on conscious and unconscious levels in the creation and recreation of human experience.

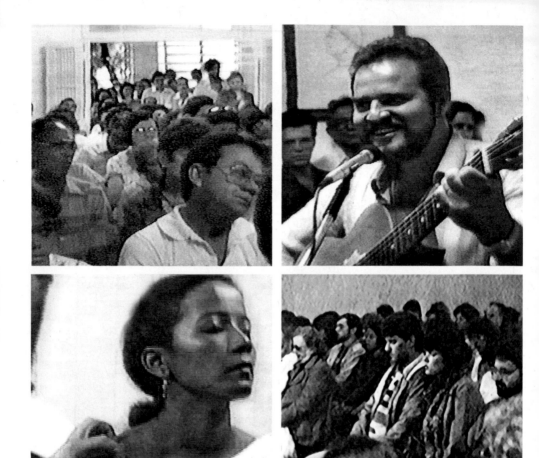

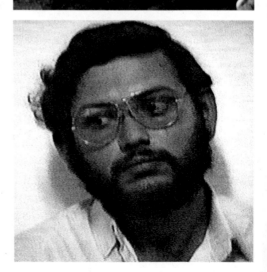

(Upper left) Patients listening to testimonials as they wait for treatment. (Upper right) Edson Queriroz entertaining waiting patients. (Middle left) Patient in trance as Edson Queiroz/Dr. Fritz inserts unwashed finger in incision in her shoulder. (Middle right) Second group of patients listening to testimonials as they wait for treatment. (Lower) Patient in trance as he waits for treatment.

CHAPTER 18

CULTURALBIOLOGY AND THE MARKETPLACE OF RELIGIONS IN BRAZIL

I was in Recife at the Centro Espírita Dr. Adolph Fritz again—not physically, but, with the help of my videotapes, field notes, memory, and whatever written material I could find, reconstructing what took place prior to the ubiquitous German spirit directing a scalpel, scissors, or needles at the first patient. I wanted to know if, as I now suspected, the patients could have been in a hypnotic trance or ASC. Dr. Fritz had argued vociferously that his patients were neither mesmerized nor hypnotized, and I had not detected anything like a formal induction process when he and other healer-mediums worked. But could something else have produced the same result? Or had sufficient time elapsed so that those waiting to see him had gone through at least one 90 to 120 minute ultradian cycle, during which they spontaneously nodded off? I wanted to know if relevant information about Kardecism's alternative reality, comparable to suggestions given by a hypnotherapist in a clinical setting, could have been transduced culturalbiologically to turn on immediate-early genes and activate endorphins and the immune and other physiological systems before the invasion of the body by the spirit with his scalpel had taken place.

One Wednesday evening, I had arrived at the center at 8:00 p.m., along with the patients and their families. We had all registered the previous weekend and had returned on Monday for the spirit to conduct what he called a triage. The majority of the people were given prescriptions for allopathic, homeopathic, herbal, and other medications, along with instructions on how they were to be taken. A smaller, second group was told that they were scheduled to have "surgery at a distance" by the spirits. Like my friend Paulo in Porto Alegre, these patients were told to go to bed under white covers, dressed in white, and to quietly read from Allan Kardec or another Spiritist writer at a specific time and date. Earlier in the week, these patients were supposed to visit a Spiritist center, receive hand passes, listen to lectures, and place glasses of water that had been "fluidified" in a special process on their dressers. At an appointed hour, they were supposed to relax, close their eyes, and go to sleep. The surgery would be performed before they were to awake several hours later and drink the water. The final group, the smallest numerically, was told to return on Wednesday to be treated in person by Edson/Fritz. The results of the triage were made available when we came to the center on Tuesday.

At 8:00 p.m. sharp the following evening, the president of the center welcomed everyone, invoked God and the spirits, and read aloud from Allan Kardec's interpretation of the Gospel. He introduced a woman who was the president of a Spiritist organization in a neighboring state. In a soft monotone, similar to that used by most of the speakers, she told the story of how she had been cured by the spirits. Suffering with a liver ailment, the exact cause of which her doctor could not diagnose, on the advice of a relative she sought aid at a Spiritist center, where a renowned spirit was treating patients through a popular medium. At that time in her life, she was not a Spiritist and knew little about Spiritist beliefs, which she thought was true for most of those listening to her. While waiting to be seen by the healer-medium, she had listened to a series of speakers expound on the Kardecist view of the universe, the dual planes of reality, and the role of spirits seeking moral advancement in both by incarnating to learn lessons, disincarnating, and incarnating once more. The woman had heard about the Kardecist view of illness and its place in the divine scheme. She knew how enlightened spirits in the other world, such as Dr. Fritz and his team, performed acts of charity by returning to this domain to treat the suffering through mediums.

The story was presented matter-of-factly. The speaker did not attempt to engage her audience, nor did she look directly at them. Furthermore, there was little inflection in her voice, and at first I was not sure that those waiting were even paying attention. When she finished, a second person told his tale of being cured by the spirits. He repeated the lecture on Spiritist cosmology and beliefs given by the previous speaker, adapting it to the specifics of his own experience with illness. His voice was flat and without inflection, as were those of the speakers to follow him. Each speaker repeated the same overview of Kardecist beliefs, modified to fit the specifics of his or her own circumstances. Time passed; the testimonials continued.

As I panned the room with my video camera and caught the expressions on the faces and the way people held their bodies of those waiting, I realized that heads were nodding rhythmically; eyelids blinked slowly and were closed over with a faraway look. Bodies were perfectly still, with fingers, hands, and legs seemingly frozen in awkward positions. Facial features were passive and slack. As I looked at the videotapes I had taken those many years before, it became clear that people in them showed the characteristics that Erickson, Rossi, and others had written about when they described patient/clients in common everyday and hypnotically facilitated trances.

The testimonials, with their emphasis on Kardec's worldview, continued for more than two hours as the patients and their guests quietly waited for Edson to arrive. It became clearer to me that the ritual actually started with the opening invocation, when everyone was exposed to the Kardecist view of the dual universe and the role played by spirits for several hours before the patients went before the medium and his guide for treatment. They each passed through at least one ultradian cycle while being exposed to the Kardecist message. The signs of them being in trance were evident.

Suddenly that night, a buzzing spread throughout the room. "The healer is here." "Edson has arrived." As people shuffled, trying to collect their thoughts, the medium, not yet embodied by the German doctor, strode to the front of the room with a guitar in his hand. For the next twenty minutes he entertained the crowd, with playing and singing reminiscent of José Carlos's performance in Fortaleza. He had a pleasant voice and appeared to be a stereotypical Brazilian who loved and made music. The words he sang contained Kardecist messages that were set to popular rhythmic strains. The atmosphere of somber reflection so characteristic of Spiritist sessions was transformed into more of a folk music concert. People cheered and applauded. Then he suddenly stopped. Edson put down his guitar and walked into a small room, where, to the reading of passages from Kardec, he went into trance and received the German doctor. An assistant called the first patient.

Lectures, readings from Kardec and other Spiritist authors, and testimonials that summarize the basic beliefs and worldview of the group precede surgeries by Spiritist healer-mediums. The highly motivated patients may have habitual patterns of association inter-rupted as they sit and listen. The information necessary for trans-duction, to activate bodily systems, is presented, and sufficient time elapses for each individual to pass through one ultradian cycle. If they did not go into trance in response to the voices of the speakers, it more than likely would happen spontaneously. Was this the key to scientifically explaining the seemingly anomalous surgeries and oth-er healings by the spirits and their mediums? Could it account, for example, for Fatima—the young woman in chapter 2 who so feared having surgery to remove the growth in her shoulder—not flinching when Edson/Fritz cut into her and extracted the grayish, infected material with his fingers? Did it also explain why those whose cor-neas were scraped to remove pterygiums and other growths did not feel pain or develop infections, even when contaminants were delib-erately introduced? Is this why Antonio's patient could be cut with a scalpel and as he bled, with his innards exposed, could continue a conversation as if he were not even aware of what was happening?

Poring over the data, I realized that the sessions at which medi-ums perform spectacular feats of healing while in trance start with indoctrination lectures followed by testimonials. But all do not last ninety minutes, the minimum time necessary for each patient to pass through one ultradian cycle. I had not observed what took place in

Fortaleza before José Carlos had turned to the first patient. Likewise, I had not observed what happened in Palmelo before Antonio received Dr. Stams and began to work. But both mediums and their spirits were able to treat patients because committed believers had made available, as charity, the conditions necessary for them to work. It was likely that they had provided speakers who presented their views of the sacred through personal stories of their own cures. But I am not sure how long those preliminary sessions lasted.

Disobsession rituals I filmed in Rio de Janeiro and Porto Alegre lasted less than ninety minutes, not long enough for all those present to go through one ultradian cycle. Consequently, not all the patients treated there and in Fortaleza and Palmelo would necessarily have entered an ASC. But those who did enter ASC had sufficient information about the other reality to transduce it and activate their bodily systems.

I was convinced that at least some of the patients did enter an ASC during the preliminary presentations. Why had Edson/Fritz and the others been so adamant about the patients being neither mesmerized nor hypnotized? One reason could be that they had not been present during the opening acts of the performances in which they were to star. The theater metaphor provides further insight. In the tradition of Europe and the Americas, those on stage—the actors—present the performance. They are separated from the audience by what in theater is known as the fourth wall. Good actors, deeply engaged in a part, take on or enter the persona of the character. Members of the audience have no reason to and do not go into trance, unless invited on stage as in the case of hypnotism. Then the volunteers are formally induced. Suggestions cause them to behave in ways that elicit laughter.

Medicine, especially surgery, follows a model of the theater (historically, the operating room was called an operating theater). Surgeons are the performers; all eyes focus on them. Their patients, like a subject brought on stage by a hypnotist, react only to what is done to them.

Spiritist healer-mediums follow the model of Western theater, only they knowingly go into trance to receive their spirit guides. The patients are members of the audience. They are not expected to be in trance, even when brought on stage. To do so would be deviating from normative cultural expectations.

In West Africa there is no symbolic wall between the parties in a performance. What we would strain to categorize as members of an audience are part of the performance. Everyone participates in a ritual. Victor Turner (1988, 1987), in addition to making explicit the way the other reality is transmitted, has shown that these social events may best be understood as performances. When Celestina de Araujo Santos, the young beautician we met in chapter 11, first went to the Casa de Vovô Maria, she sat separated from those at the front of the room. Once the gira began, she and everyone else was swept up by the music. The mãe-de-santo might have made a mental note of it, but had Celestina entered an ASC and received a spirit before having any special preparation, no one would have been surprised.

The drumming, singing, chanting, and dancing at African-derived rituals in Brazil provide sufficient rhythmic, auditory, and other stimulation to induce an ASC in many who attend them, even for the first time. Since the rituals go on for hours, often into the early light of morning, there is sufficient time for everyone present to pass through at least one ultradian cycle. Enough time elapses that the information contained in the ritual interrupts habitual patterns of association.

Celestina and the other first-timers may not have initially shared the belief system of their Umbanda hosts, but they were there because they had been told, and wanted to believe, that the pomba gira and other spirits could and would help them. They had seen and been embraced by the orixás/saints and had watched a young Antonio be "transformed" before their eyes into the aged preto velho. There was no need for details about the belief system. There was enough convincing information about Umbanda's sacred reality that if a newcomer did enter an ASC, Umbanda's beliefs could be transduced to activate bodily mechanisms that would begin the healing process, a process that would continue after he or she left the center.

When Celestina returned for the trabalho, the special ritual Mãe Edna recommended, the repetitive music and drumming could have brought the knowledge she had learned at the previous session, and had heard from her cousin in the weeks before and after, into her working memory to be transduced and to again stimulate her body's responses, accounting for her mysterious recovery. And the same process would explain the many cures reported by people who turn to other religions. Ruth Landes ([1947] 1994:75) tells us of a Bahian colleague who said that the possession behavior of participants in the African-derived religions could be "attributed to nothing more abnormal than hypnotism." Another colleague told her, "He stuck pins into those priestesses when they were dancing, and they never felt the pain. He passed objects before their eyes, and the pupils never focused." Many of the participants in Afro-Brazilian rituals enter ASC while being told about the ability of the orixás to help them. The transduction of this information, under these circumstances, can account for the cures and other benefits reported.

The *cultos,* as the lengthy ritual services of many of the IURD and other evangelical churches in Brazil are called, begin with rhythmic singing, hand clapping, and foot stomping to the beat of electric guitars. Those who come for the first time are encouraged to, and often do, enter into trance to incorporate their orixá, exu, or other evil spirits so that they may be exorcised and the newcomer liberated. These entities are considered to be forms of the devil. While in trance, the highly motivated visitors listen to the pastor; invited members of the congregation give testimonials on how the Holy Spirit cured them of illness or helped them turn their lives around. The newcomers do not share the epistemology and worldview of the church community when they arrive. But the information presented is sufficient for it to be transduced into someone in an ASC, so that the bodies of some of those suffering begin to heal naturally, explaining the many cases reported in the seemingly never-ending testimonials given in evangelical churches and on radio and television. Although the evangelicals come from the Western tradition, their ritual performances are more like West African practice, in that the members of the congregation are not separated from the pastor and others "on stage" by a fourth wall.

Romeiros, who make pilgrimages to the shrines of Catholic saints, do not participate in a group ritual when they make their promessas, which are offered in solitude. Certainly, Fatima reported that she prayed with conviction and intensity for a long time when she asked St. Francis to intercede on her behalf and help her when she hurt her leg. I do not know how long it took her to complete the vow, or if she or any of the others fulfilling their obligations in Canindé entered an

ASC at the time. Certainly, all who make vows to the saints are highly motivated. Thinking about what she had learned at church services as a child, and the many stories she had been told about the way the saint had helped others, may have helped move the relevant information to current memory. Being in an ASC so that the culturalbiological process could work would explain the many "miracles" that bring Brazilians and others to places like Canindé to fulfill their vows.

This book began with descriptions of surgeries by Kardecist-Spiritist healer-mediums who, when incorporated by their guides, cut into patients with surgical scalpels, unclean knives, scissors, and even an electric saw. They inserted needles into all parts of the body and introduced dirty fingers and other contaminants while removing growths and infected material. The patients reported feeling little or no pain, did not develop infections or other complications, and recovered. In another form of therapy, a group leader sent mediums to the other world to incorporate spirits, with whose help he reconstructed events in a past life of a patient to precipitate a cure. Since both sets of events cannot be explained in terms of commonsense understandings based on conventional medical science, the rational, intellectual Kardecists used them to proselytize, arguing that only their view of reality can explain what the patients experienced and what their loved ones and others witnessed. Since the surgeries and healings happened and were inexplicable in terms of everything those present knew and believed, their only choice was to accept Kardecism, join one of its centers, and contribute to its agenda of helping those in need as charity.

Part II of the book showed that other religious groups in Brazil offered healing by the spirits or supernatural(s) to gain converts. The success stories are also inexplicable in terms of conventional medical science. Each group promised a cure or other help for the needy. Kardecism, popular Catholicism, Umbanda, Candomblé, the other African-derived groups, as well as Pentecostal Protestantism, were seen to be providers of services, with healing by their specific forms of the supernatural being paramount, in a competitive marketplace in which consumers shopped, going from one ritual performance to the next until finding satisfaction. The customers paid for their purchases by converting and affiliating with the group that had helped them. While this analysis enabled us to understand the proselytizing activities of religious groups in Brazil and the regular movement of individuals from one religion to another, it was in part III that I returned to the healing events that seem inexplicable in terms of conventional medical science.

The model proposed elaborates on work conducted at the forefront of science in fields such as neuroscience, psychoneuroimmunology, and psychobiology. Building primarily on the writings of Ernest L. Rossi, I suggest that culture, as information, often held implicitly in a group's sacred understandings but made explicit during religious rituals, could function analogously to a therapist's suggestions made to a patient in a hypnotically induced trance. Furthermore, under the right circumstances, this information could be transduced to become part of the communication flow within an individual organism, turning on or off immediate-early genes and physiological systems that contribute to healing. Suffering individuals participating in a religious ritual, even if they do not share the beliefs and epistemology of the group, could enter into an ASC—brought on by singing, drumming, dancing, hand clapping, or the continuous droning of uninflected voices—during which the belief that spirits or another form of the supernatural could cure them would become part of the expanding view of therapy and healing.

When the sacred beliefs of a specific culture or religion are added, as information, to the new paradigm for medicine and healing, we have an explanation for the anomalous events described. Dr. Fritz, St. Francis, Oxalá, the pomba gira, and the Holy Ghost may or may not actually cure. However, the belief in any one of them, and their ability to relieve pain and suffering, may cure when it is placed as information in the working memory of a participant in a religious ritual. In an ASC, that information may be transduced, via the brain, to become part of the communication flow. This in turn may release the body's own painkillers (endorphins) and activate the immune and other systems, analogous to the way suggestions in hypnotically facilitated therapy work.[52]

The model does not tell us if a specific individual will enter an ASC during a ritual and transduce the beliefs presented to receive the promised results. Some individuals will be cured, but some will not. The ritual of a group chosen may not provide the hoped-for outcome. Not finding relief in Umbanda, for example, a sufferer will try Candomblé. If unsuccessful there, a Pentecostal church might be next, or perhaps a vow to a saint, or a visit to a Spiritist center. But even if the sufferer finds success and joins the group that provided it, culturalbiology might not be repeated in the event of a new problem. When another mishap befalls the individual, the process begins again. This time he or she might not enter an ASC and have the belief in a supernatural transduced to activate the needed bodily responses. As long as religious groups in Brazil continue to offer healing to gain converts, and people in need cannot be helped all the time, the religious marketplace will persevere.

Postscript

In the novel *When the Sleeper Awakes,* written at the end of the nineteenth century, Graham, H. G. Wells's protagonist, when he opens his eyes in the early years of the twenty-second century, is informed that "some very interesting developments [had taken place during the preceding centuries] in the art of hypnotism." To his surprise, Graham learns that hypnosis *"had largely superseded drugs, antiseptics and anesthetics in medicine."* As a result, Wells tells us, "A real enlargement of human faculty seemed to have been effected" (Wells [1899] 2000:274; italics added).

Wells's prediction that hypnotically facilitated therapy would supersede drugs, antiseptics, and anesthetics is only beginning to be appreciated and applied in the healing practices of Western society. Many of the premises of the new paradigm, in which cultural beliefs, now understood as information analogous to suggestions, are found in the ritual healing practices of Brazil's popular religions, as part of the communication flow that turns on the body's responses. Spiritist healer-mediums, pais- and mães-de-santo of Candomblé and Umbanda, and evangelical pastors, like "traditional" and "alternative" healers everywhere, are doing what Wells only imagined. Although it is in the laboratories and clinics where the new framework is being advanced and tested, perhaps anthropology, with its understanding of culture, has a contribution to make to the new vision. I hope my colleagues and their students will join me in the pursuit of this new adventure.

NOTES

1. This seemed to be related to contributions by Claude Lévi-Strauss (1963) and other anthropologists regarding the role played by symbols and their meanings in illness, and its cure cross-culturally.

2. Placebo surgeries are not new in medicine. In 1939 Freischi developed a procedure to increase blood flow to the myocardium of angina patients. Twenty years later, in a trial of seventeen patients, nine were anesthetized and got incisions, but nothing else. The placebo surgeries worked as well as the actual surgeries (Kent 2002; Cobb et al. 1959). Placebo surgeries also have been done on patients with Parkinson's disease in place of operations to implant stem cells from aborted human fetuses (Kent 2002; Freed et al. 2001).

3. Today we would say human beings.

4. St. Ignatius is also the primary spirit received by João Teixeira de Farias, a healer-medium from Abadiânia, another town in the interior of the state of Goiás. João is popular in Brazil and the United States, which he visits periodically. He is known in English as John of God.

5. See Greenfield (2006) for information on the personal life of the doctor.

6. A sample of the surgeries described in this chapter may be seen in Greenfield and Gray (1988).

7. He was pointing to a pterygium, a raised, wedge-shaped growth of the conjunctiva that is most common among those who live in the tropics.

8. It has since changed its name to the Committee for Skeptical Inquiry (CSI).

9. Studying another healer, a team including Brazilian medical doctors and surgeons observed and took samples of materials cut during surgeries. The team concluded that the surgeries were "actual procedures and the extracted tissues were compatible with the body region from where they were removed. No evidence of fraud was detected" (Krippner 2008:24).

10. James Braid, a Scotsman practicing medicine in Manchester in the 1830s and 1840s, is generally credited with inventing "the word 'hypnosis'" after hearing a lecture by one of Mesmer's disciples (Inglis 1989:61). Gravitz (1984), however, claims that the term *hypnotisme* was coined in the first decade of the 1800s in France. Ironically, as Braid and others in England and France were experimenting with painless surgeries on hypnotized patients, laughing gas, supplemented by chloroform, was being introduced as an anesthetic (Inglis 1989:59).

11. The commission, writes St. Clair (1971:90), "pronounced that it was all in the patients' minds and 'magnetism' did not exist."

12. Some of the therapies offered at Spiritist centers, such as the surgeries, can complement or be an alternative to conventional medicine.

13. These demographics did not differ significantly from those I observed at centers where patients waited to be treated by José Carlos, Edson, Antonio, and Mauricio. While at times poor black people were more numerous (as they are in the general population), especially when the healer-medium was visiting a center in a major metropolitan area, Kardecism still tends to attract larger numbers from the middle and upper classes, who are light skinned and better educated.

14. This group has reached out atypically to encompass Umbanda and its spirits (see chapter 11).

15 Brazilian religions are highly syncretic, with each frequently

adopting features of the others. It is not unusual to find elements from Umbanda and Candomblé employed by usually middle-class European Kardecists like those of the Casa do Jardim. Likewise, Candomblé and Umbanda may at times seem to envision their Africa deities as if they were Christian saints. In addition, Brazilian religions also are quite porous, with individuals changing their affiliations fairly regularly.

16. The disobsession contains all the key elements in what Harrington (2008:36) calls the exorcism drama, which has been played out regularly in Christian history.

17. These, since they are based primarily on Bezerra de Menezes's reading of Kardec's interpretation of mental illness, are alternative rather than complementary therapies, as Dr. Hervé made clear when he explained to the first patient that her symptoms could be treated adequately by conventional medicine.

18. Starting in the Paraíba Valley between Rio de Janeiro and São Paulo, coffee cultivation moved rapidly across the latter and westward into Paraná.

19. Examples are the densely populated societies encountered on the Indian subcontinent, in Southeast Asia, and in tropical Africa.

20. The large and ever-growing number of popular saints selected by the people created a dilemma for the church and its administrative hierarchy. Although veneration of saints undercut the emphasis the church wished to place on the divine Trinity as the focus of the religion, the saints did serve as role models. The stories of these exceptional human beings, elaborated in myth, served to teach the virtues that church leaders wished to instill in followers. Rather than downplay the cult of the saints, the church chose instead to take control of the saint-making process (Woodward 1990). Starting in 1234, the right to determine whom God had chosen and elevated from among the once living was reserved to the papacy alone. However, Roman Catholics today still worship many more saints than those officially recognized by the Vatican.

21. He is said to have written to the three brothers who owned the land, asking them to donate it as a patrimony for a church. When

they refused, the supernatural intervention that has come to be associated with the site reportedly began. One of the brothers took sick and died shortly thereafter. Then, following a brief illness, a second brother also died. When the third brother took ill, he immediately made the donation Madeiros had requested. He reportedly recovered as mysteriously as he had become ill and his brothers had died (Greenfield 1989, 1987b).

22. The Bight of Benin runs some 450 miles from the mouth of the Volta River to the mouth of the Niger.

23 Brazil has the largest Japanese population outside Japan.

24. In a national survey conducted in the mid-1990s, Pierucci and Prandi (1996) found that in terms of race, 51 percent of the followers of Afro-Brazilian religions in Brazil were white. Another 29 percent were *pardos* (mixed race), and only 18 percent were *negros*. For Umbanda alone, the figures were 57 percent white, 27 percent pardos, and 15 percent black. For Candomblé, 40 percent of practitioners were white, 33 percent pardo, and 24 percent black (Oro 1999:45, n. 17).

25. The American Bible Society hired the Reverend James C. Fletcher to superintend shipments of Bibles to Brazil between 1854 and 1856. The Congregational Church, in the person of Robert Reid Kalley, came to Rio de Janeiro in 1855, and the Presbyterians arrived in 1859 (Read 1965:180–256; Williams, Bartless and Miller 1955:756, 777; Crabtree 1937:28–30).

26. Which in turn was derived from the teaching of John Wesley (1703–91), founder of Methodism.

27. Others acknowledge Charles P. Parham, a white preacher, and his Bethel Bible School in Topeka, Kansas, as the beginning of the movement (see Kendrick 1961). Seymour first studied and then split with Parham. Similar movements, all with comparable messages, appeared in the same period elsewhere in the United States, Puerto Rico, and Mexico.

28. A story says that one day, when the immigrants were speaking in tongues, the word *para* was repeated several times. Looking it up in a world atlas, the men discovered that Pará was the name of a Brazilian state. Interpreting this as a prophecy, they gathered

their money and effects and departed for a missionary trip to its capital (Curry n.d.:75).

29. The latter, with its strong presence in São Paulo, which was receiving large numbers of immigrants from Europe, had 36,644 devotees by 1936, the first year statistics were available. The AD reported a modest 14,000 members six years earlier. By 1950 the CC had mushroomed to 132,297, with the AD estimating 120,000 one year earlier.

30 Curry (n.d.) claims that the foreign missionaries never understood Brazilian society because they saw it through the postfeudal eyes of the "rural-urban" dichotomy.

31. Then there's the story, reported by Curry (1968:258), of the aged mother of a pastor of the Pentecostal Church. Although living with her minister son, on whom she was dependent, she remained Catholic. Then she took drastically sick with what she believed would be her last illness. When she recovered, following the prayers and attentions of the Protestant congregation, she completed the *promessa* she had made and converted.

32 An additional 38.4 percent earned between one and two minimum wages (Fleischer, March 27–April 21, 2006). Brazilians think in terms of earnings per month instead of per year. The unit of currency at the time this book was published was the *real* (plural *reais;* written R$). It was put into use in 1994 to replace the cruzeiro. One U.S. dollar was equal to approximately 1.7 reais in 2008.

33 The administration of President Luiz Ignácio "Lula" da Silva has made a concerted effort to create jobs and decrease unemployment. In 2007, for example, 1,617,392 new positions (with benefits) were created, 31 percent more that in 2006 and more than the record 1,523,276 new jobs generated in 2004 (Fleischer, January 12–18, 2008). Most of the new work opportunities pay the minimum wage. However, average income has declined slightly because an increasing number of these positions are not full-time (Fleischer, January 15–51, 2005). Industrial employment increased by 2.2 percent between 2006 and 2007. Average industrial income was up 5.4 percent in the same period and up

9.7 percent since 2004 (Fleischer, February 2–22, 2008). The new jobs, combined with the sizable number of people who have given up seeking employment, have led to a reduction in the official unemployment rate.

34 Meanwhile, according to Pochmann (cited in Fleischer, January 24–February 4, 2005), in the last two decades of the twentieth century the number of wealthy families increased by 500,000, to 2.4 percent from 1.8 percent of the population, and now control one-third of the wealth.

35. It is not uncommon to find members of a single family or household affiliated with different, seemingly contradictory faiths.

36. According to a 1998 study on sexual behavior and perceptions of HIV/AIDS, reported in Almeida and Monteiro (2001), 26 percent of a sample population from all over Brazil changed religion. For mobility between religions, see Prandi (1996) and Fernandes et al (1998).

37. Pert (1997:18) puts it more bluntly when she writes that Descartes "was forced to make a turf deal with the Pope in order to get the human bodies he needed for dissection. Descartes agreed he wouldn't have anything to do with the soul, the mind or emotions—those aspects of the human experience under the virtually exclusive jurisdiction of the church at the time—if he could claim the physical realm as his own."

38. Referring to all aspects of human thought, feeling, and understanding, including beliefs in spirits and the supernatural.

39. Gravity also has no length, breadth, or thickness. It can be defined only, in a procedure considered invalid since the end of the medieval period, by stating what characteristics it has, which are those consciously attributed to it by the members of a scientific community when, for example, they wish to explain observations made on solar phenomena.

40. According to Pert and her colleagues,

> "Many of these informal substances are neuropeptides, originally studied in other contexts ... most, if not all, alter behavior and mood states. ... We now realize that their signal specificity resides in receptors (distinct classes of recognition molecules).

... Rather precise brain distribution patterns for many neuro-peptide receptors have been determined. A number of brain loci, many within emotion-mediating brain areas, are enriched with many types of neuropeptide receptors suggesting a convergence of information at these 'nodes.' Additionally, neuro-peptide receptors occur on middle cells of the immune systems; monocytes can chemotax to numerous neuropeptides via processes shown by structure-activity analysis to be mediated by distinct receptors indistinguishable from those found in the brain. Neuropeptides and their receptors thus join the brain, glands, and immune system in a network of communication between brain and body, probably representing the biochemical substrate of emotion" (Pert et al. 1985:820s).

41. Transduction is the process by which information is transformed from one energy medium into another. A microphone, for example, transduces the sound waves we produce when we talk or sing into electrical impulses; loudspeakers transduce electrical impulses into sound waves we receive via our ears. The technology at the grocery store's checkout counter transforms bar codes on purchases into laser light reflections, then electrical impulses, and finally a mechanically imprinted itemized bill.

42. Nørretranders (1998:124) observes that this "has been known for almost forty years, yet remains relatively unnoticed even though it constitutes one of the most important testimonies we have about what it means to be human."

43. This might be what Jungians are referring to when they speak of the collective unconscious.

44. This may be thought of in Geertz's (1973:93) sense as a model *of* reality becoming a model *for* (real) behavior, independent of an individual actor's conscious awareness and intentionality.

45. Unfortunately, he adds as a caveat:

"Clinical investigations have usually not been designed in ways permitting unambiguous conclusions about the manner in which mind has influenced body. Often it is not clear whether the outcome was a result of hypnosis, relaxation, education, emotional support, or expectancy" (Holroyd 1992:207–08).

46. It is important to note that most of the professional training of these students is in psychology.

47. This was in spite of the claims of Milton Erickson, founder of the American Society of Clinical Hypnosis, that everyone regularly enters into what he called common everyday trance (Rossi and Rossi 1996:131–32).

48. For a review of the literature on altered states of consciousness and religious behavior, see Winkelman (1997).

49. Rodgers (2006:281) observes that "placebos can be as much as 70 percent effective in the treatment of illness."

50. Elsewhere Rossi (2001:156) contends that it happens most significantly in special moments, when "a habitual pattern of association is interrupted," as when patients step before an embodied Kardecist healer-medium with scalpel in hand, a possessed *pai-* or *mãe-de-santo*, or a zealous evangelical pastor.

51. When the information is negative, the outcome may be detrimental, as in the case of spells, curses, and even voodoo death.

52. Alternatively, individuals who already share the belief system of the group performing a ritual can bring the belief in the ability of its supernatural(s) from implicit to working memory, and if they enter an ASC can achieve the same results. In this way, the transformation imagery proposed by medical anthropology is articulated with psychology and biology.

REFERENCES

ABC. 2005. "Is 'John of God' a Healer or a Charlatan?" *Primetime Live.* February 10. http://abcnews.go.com/Health/Primetime/story?id=482292&page=1.

Acquarone, Francisco. 1982. *Bezerra de Menezes: O Medico dos Pobres.* 6th edition. São Paulo: Editora Aliança.

Ader, Robert, and Nicholas Cohen. 1991. *Psychoneuroimmunology.* 2nd edition. San Diego: Academic Press.

Aijmer, G. 1995. *Syncretism and the Commerce of Symbols.* Göteborg, Sweden: Institute for Advanced Studies in Social Anthropology, Göteborg University.

Akstein, David. 1977. Socio-cultural Basis of Terpsichoretrancetherapy. *American Journal of Clinical Hypnosis* 19:221–25.

———. 1973. Terpsichoretrancetherapy: A New Hypnotherapeutic Method. *International Journal of Clinical and Experimental Hypnosis* 21:131–43.

———. 1965. The Induction of Hypnosis in the Light of Reflexology. *American Journal of Clinical Hypnosis* 8:281–300.

Almeida, Alexander M., Tatiana M. Almeida, Ângela M. Gollner, and Stanley Krippner. n.d. A Hystocytopathological Study of Mediumistic Surgery. Unpublished manuscript.

Almeida, Alexander M., Tatiana M. Almeida, and Ângela M. Gollner. 2000. Cirurgia Espiritual: Uma Investigação. *Revista Associação Medica Brasileira* 46(3):194–200.

Almeida, Ronaldo de, and Paula Monteiro. 2001. *Trásito Religioso no Brasil.* São Paulo Perspectiva 15:3.

Anderson, Allan. 2004. *An Introduction to Pentecostalism.* Cambridge, England: Cambridge University Press.

Armstrong, Karen. 2000. *The Battle for God.* New York: Ballantine Books.

Atkinson, R. L, R. C. Atkinson, E. E. Smith, and D. J. Bem. 1990. *Introduction to Psychology.* New York: Harcourt Brace Jovanovich.

Azzi, R. 1978. *O Catolicismo Popular no Brasil.* Petrópolis, Brazil: Editora Vozes.

Bailey, C. H., D. Bartsch, and E. R. Kandel. 1996. Toward a Molecular Definition of Long-term Memory Storage. *Proceedings of the National Academy of Sciences of the United States of America* 93:13445–52.

Barber, T. X. 1999. A Comprehensive Three Dimensional Theory of Hypnosis. In *Clinical Hypnosis and Self Regulation.* I. Kirsch, A. Capafons, E. Cardena-Beulna, and S. Amigo, eds., pp. 21–48. Washington, DC: American Psychological Association.

———— 1984. Changing "Unchangeable" Bodily Processes by (Hypnotic) Suggestions: A New Look at Hypnosis, Cognitions, Imagining, and the Mind-body Problem. In *Imagination and Healing.* A. A. Sheikh., ed., pp. 69–127. Farmingdale, NY: Baywood Publishing Company.

Barreto, Adalberto de P. 1986. A Romaria e a Doença. Paper presented at the meetings of the Latin American Studies Association, Boston.

————. n.d. Exvotos: Os Milagres dos Santos. Unpublished manuscript.

Basso, E. 1985. *A Musical View of the Universe: Kalapalo Myth and Ritual Performance.* Philadelphia: University of Pennsylvania Press.

Bastide, Roger. 1978. *The African Religions of Brazil: Toward a Sociology of the Interpenetration of Civilizations.* H. Sebba, trans. Baltimore: Johns Hopkins University Press.

————. 1951. Religion and the Church in Brazil. In *Brazil: Portrait of Half a Continent.* T. L. Smith and A. Marchant, eds., pp. 334–49. New York: Dryden.

Beattie, J. 1964. *Other Cultures: Aims, Methods and Achievements in Social Anthropology.* New York: Free Press.

Black, S. 1969. *Mind and Body.* London: Kimber.

Bloch, M. 1991. Language, Anthropology and Cognitive Science. *Man* 26(2):183–98.

Boas, Franz. 1966. *Kwakiutl Ethnography.* Helen Codere, ed. Chicago: University of Chicago Press.

References

Bogoras, W. [1904–09] 1979. The Chukchee. In *Reader in Comparative Religion: An Anthropological Approach*. 4th edition. W. Lessa and E. Vogt, eds., pp. 302–07. New York: Harper and Row.

Bonewits, I. [1971] 1993. *Real Magic: An Introductory Treatise on the Basic Principles of Yellow Magic*. York Beach, ME: Samuel Weisner Inc.

Bourguignon, Erika. 1976. *Possession*. San Francisco: Chandler and Sharp.

———. 1973. *Religion, Altered States of Consciousness and Social Change*. Columbus: Ohio State University Press.

———. 1968. *A Cross-cultural Study of Dissociational States: Final Report*. Columbus, OH: Research Foundation.

Bourguignon, Erika, and T. Evascu. 1977. Altered States of Consciousness within a General Evolutionary Perspective: A Holocultural Analysis. *Behavior Science Research* 12:197–216.

Bowers, K. 1977. Hypnosis: An Informational Approach. *Annals of the New York Academy of Sciences* 296:222–37.

———. 1966. Hypnotic Behavior: The Differentiation of Trance and Demand Characteristic Variables. *Journal of Abnormal Psychology* 71:42–51.

Fleischer, David. 2004–08. "Brazil Focus." *Brazil Institute*. *http://www.wilson center.org/index.cfm?topic_id=1419&fuseaction=Topics.home*.

The Brazilians. 2004–2005. "Miséria Atinge 27 Millões de Crianças Brasileiras." December–January.

Brown, D. P. 1992. Clinical Hypnosis Research since 1986. In *Contemporary Hypnosis Research*. E. Fromm and M. R. Nash, eds., pp. 427–58. New York: Guilford Press.

Brown, D. P., and E. Fromm. 1987. *Hypnosis and Behavioral Medicine*. Hillsdale, NJ: Erlbaum Associates.

Brown, Diana DeG. [1986] 1994. *Umbanda: Religion and Politics in Urban Brazil*. New York: Columbia University Press.

Brown, Peter. 1981. *The Cult of the Saints*. Chicago: University of Chicago Press.

Caravalho, Margarida de. 1995. A Healing Journey in Brazil: A Case Study in Spiritual Surgery. *Journal of the Society for Psychical Research* 60:161–67.

———. 1996. An Eclectic Approach to Group Healing in Sao Paulo, Brazil: A Pilot Study. *Journal of the Society for Psychical Research* 61:243–50.

REFERENCES

Carroll, James. 2001. *Constantine's Sword: The Church and the Jews: A History.* Boston: Houghton Mifflin.

Castés, M., I. Hagel, M. Palanque, P. Canelones, A. Carao, and N. R. Lynch. 1999. Immunological Changes Associated with Clinical Improvement of Asthmatic Children Subjected to Psychosocial Intervention. *Brain, Behavior, and Immunity* 13:1–13.

Cavalcante, Antonio Mourão. 1987. As Festas da Festa. *Diario de Noticias,* October 11.

Cavalcanti, Maria Laura. 1983. *O Mundo Invisível: Cosmologia, Sistema Ritualm e Noção de Pessoa no Espiritismo.* Rio de Janeiro: Zahar Editoras.

Cesar, Waldo. 2000. Daily Life and Transcendence. In *Pentecostalism and the Future of Christian Churches,* by Richard Shaull and Waldo Cesar, pp. 3–111. Grand Rapids, MI: William B. Eerdmans Publishing Co.

Chaves, J. F., and T. X. Barber. 1974. Cognative Strategies, Experimental Modeling, and Expectation in the Attenuation of Pain. *Journal of Abnormal Psychology* 83:356–63.

Chestnut, R. Andrew. 1997. *Born Again in Brazil: The Pentecostal Boom and Pathogens of Poverty.* New Brunswick: Rutgers University Press.

Cobb, L. A., G. I. Thomas, D. H. Dillard, et al. 1959. An Evaluation of Internal Mammary Artery Ligation by a Double-Blind Technique. *New England Journal of Medicine* 260:1115.

Cohen, Emma. 2007. *The Mind Possessed: The Cognition of Spirit Possession in an Afro-Brazilian Religious Tradition.* Oxford: Oxford University Press.

Corten, André. 1999. *Pentecostalism in Brazil: Emotion of the Poor and Theological Romanticism.* Arianne Dorval, trans. New York: St. Martin's Press.

Cousins, Norman. 1986. Foreword. In *The Healer Within: The New Medicine of the Mind and Body,* by S. Locke and D. Colligan. New York: E. P. Dutton.

Crabtree, A. R. 1937. *História dos Batistes do Brasil: Até o Ano de 1906.* Rio de Janeiro: Casa Publicadora Batista.

Crick, F. H. C. 1958. On Protein Synthesis. Symposium of the Society for Experimental Biology 12:138–63.

Crosby, Alfred W. [1986] 1993. *Ecological Imperialism.* New York: Cambridge University Press.

———. 1972. *The Columbian Exchange: Biological and Cultural Consequences of 1492.* Westport, CT: Greenwood Press.

References

Curry, Donald Edward. 1968. Lusiada: An Anthropological Study of the Growth of Protestantism in Brazil. PhD dissertation, Columbia University, New York.

——. n.d. Political and Economic Implications of the Growth of Protestantism in Brazil: With a Critique of the Thesis of Max Weber. First draft of 1968 PhD dissertation.

D'Andrade, Roy. 1995. *The Development of Cognitive Anthropology*. Cambridge: Cambridge University Press.

Dantas, Beatriz G. 1988. *Vovó Nagô e Papai Branco: Usos e Abusos da África no Brasil*. Rio de Janeiro: Edições Graal Ltda.

——. 1982. Repensando a Pureza de Nagô. *Religião e Sociedade* 8:5–20.

Dantzer, R. 1997. Stress and Immunity: What Have We Learned from Psychoneuroimmunology. *Acta Physiol Scand Suppl* 640:43–46.

Descartes, René. [1637, 1641] 1980. *Discourse on Method and Meditations on First Philosophy*. D. A. Cress, trans. Indianapolis: Hackett.

Dhabhar, F. S., and B. S. McEwen. 1996. Stress-induced Enhancement of Antigen-specific Cell-mediated Immunity. *Journal of Immunology* 156:2608–15.

Dhabhar, F. S., A. H. Miller, B. S. McEwen, and R. L. Spencer. 1995. Effects of Stress on Immune Cell Distribution. *Journal of Immunology* 154:5511–27.

Diamond, Jared. 1997. *Guns, Germs, and Steel: The Fates of Human Societies*. New York: W. W. Norton and Company.

Dow, James. 1986. Universal Aspects of Symbolic Healing: A Theoretical Synthesis. *American Anthropologist* 88:56–69.

Eliade, M. 1976. *Myths, Dreams and Mysteries: The Encounter between Contemporary Faiths and Archaic Reality*. London: Collins.

Ewin, D. M. 1984. Hypnosis in Surgery and Anesthesia. In *Clinical Hypnosis: A Multidisciplinary Approach*. W. C. Wester and A. H. Smith, eds., pp. 210–35. Philadelphia: Lippincott.Fernandes, Rubem, Pierre Sanchis, Octávio Velho, Leandro Piquet, Cecília Mariz, and Clara Mafra. 1998. *Novo Nacimento: os Evangélicos em Casa, na Política e na Igreja*. Rio de Janeiro: Mauad.

Fernandez, James, ed. 1991. *Beyond Metaphor: The Theory of Tropes in Anthropology*. Stanford, CA: Stanford University Press.

——. 1986. *Persuasions and Performances: The Play of Tropes in Culture*. Bloomington: Indiana University Press.

Ferreira, Julio Andrade. 1959. *História da Igreja Presbeteriana do Brasil*. São Paulo: Casa Editôra Presbiteriana.

References

Fleischer, David. 2004–08. "Brazil Focus." *Brazil Institute. http://www.wilson center.org/index.cfm?topic_id=1419&fuseaction=Topics.home.*

Fonseca, Alexandre B. 2003. Igreja Universal: Um Império Midiático. In *Igreja Universal do Reino de Deus: Novos Conquistadors da Fé.* Ari Pedro Oro, André Corten, and Jean-Pierre Dozon, organizers, pp. 259–80. São Paulo: Editora Paulinas.

Franco, Divaldo Pereira. 1979. *Obsession.* Dictated by the Spirit Manoel Philomena de Miranda. Ely J. Donato and Herminio C. Miranda, trans. Salvador, Brazil: Centro da Redenção.

Frazer, James G. [1911–15] 1922. *The Golden Bough: A Study in Magic and Religion.* 12 vols. 3rd edition. London: Macmillan.

Frecska, E., and Z. Kulcsar. 1989. Social Bonding in the Modulation of the Physiology of Ritual Trance. *Ethos* 17(1):70–87.

Freed, C. R., P. E. Greene, R. E. Breeze, et al. 2001. Transplantation of Embryonic Dopamine Neurons for Severe Parkinson's Disease. *New England Journal of Medicine* 344(10):710.

Freston, Paul. 1993. Protestantes e Política no Brasil: da Constituente ao Impeachment. PhD dissertation, Universidade Estadual de Campinas.

Freyre, Gilberto. 1964. *Masters and the Slaves.* S. Putnam, trans. New York: Alfred A. Knopf.

Fuller, John. 1974. *Arigo: Surgeon of the Rusty Knife.* New York: Crowell.

Fuller, Robert C. 1982. *Mesmerism and the American Cure of Souls.* Philadelphia: University of Pennsylvania Press.

Furtado, Celso. 1963. *The Economic Growth of Brazil: A Survey from Colonial to Modern Times.* Berkeley: University of California Press.

Gauld, Alan. 1992. *A History of Hypnotism.* Cambridge: Cambridge University Press.

Geertz, Clifford. 1973. *The Interpretation of Cultures.* New York: Basic Books.

Gill, M. M., and M. Brenman. 1959. *Hypnosis and Related States: Psychoanalytic Studies in Regression.* New York: International Universities Press.

Giobellina Brumana, Fernando and Elda G. Martinez. 1989. *Spirits from the Margin: Umbanda in São Paulo.* Uppsala, Sweden: Acta Universitatis Upsaliensus.

Glaser, R., S. Kennedy, W. Lafuse, R. Bonneau, C. Speicher, J. Hillhouse, and J. Kiecolt-Glaser. 1990. Psychological Stress-induced Modulation of Interleukin 2 Receptor Gene Expression and Interleukin 2 Production in Peripheral Blood Leukocytes. *Archive of General Psychiatry* 47:707–12.

References

Glaser, R., W. Lafuse, R. Bonneau, C. Atkinson, and J. Kiecolt-Glaser. 1993. Stress-associated Modulation of Proto-oncogene Expression in Human Peripheral Blood Leukocytes. *Behavioral Neuroscience* 107:525–29.

Gonsalkorale, W. M., L. A. Houghton, and P. J. Whorwell. 2002. Hypnotherapy in Irritable Bowel Syndrome: A Large Scale Audit of a Clinical Service with Examination of Factors Influencing Responsiveness. *American Journal of Gastroenterology* 97:954–61.

Gonsalkorale, W. M., V. Miller, A. Afzal, et al. 2003. Long Term Benefits of Hypnotherapy for Irritable Bowel Syndrome. *Gut* 52(11):1623–29.

Gonsalkorale, W. M., B. B. Toner, and P. J. Whorwell. 2004. Cognitive Change in Patients Undergoing Hypnotherapy for Irritable Bowel Syndrome. *Journal of Psychosomatic Research* 56(3):271–78.

Goodman, Felicitas D. 1988. *Ecstasy, Ritual and Alternate Reality: Religion in a Pluralistic World*. Bloomington: Indiana University Press.

Gravitz, Melvin. 1984. Origins of the Term Hypnosis Prior to Braid. *American Journal of Clinical Hypnosis* 27:107–10.

Greenfield, Sidney M. 2006. Dr. Fritz: Myth, Man and Spirit Guide. Paper presented at the session the Social Lives of Spirits at the 105th Annual Meetings of the American Anthropological Association, San Jose, California, November 15–19.

———. 2004. Treating the Sick with a Morality Play: The Kardecist-Spiritist Disobession in Brazil. *Social Analysis* 48(2):174–94.

———. 2003. Can Supernaturals Really Heal? *Anthropological Forum* 13:151–58.

———. 2002. The Pragmatics of Conversion in the Brazilian Religious Marketplace. In *Contemporary Cultures and Societies of Latin America*. Dwight Heath, ed., pp. 490–96. Prospect Heights, IL: Waveland Press.

———. 1997. The Patients of Dr. Fritz: Assessments of Treatment by a Brazilian Spiritist Healer. *Journal of the Society for Psychical Research* 61: 372–83.

———. 1995. *Spirits, Medicine, and Charity: A Brazilian Woman's Cure for Cancer*. Video documentary. Milwaukee: Media Resource Department, University of Wisconsin-Milwaukee.

———. 1994. Descendants of European Immigrants in Southern Brazil as Participants and Heads of Afro-Brazilian Religious Centers. *Ethnic and Racial Studies* 17(4):684–700.

———. 1993. Legacies from the Past and Transitions to a "Healed" Future in Brazilian Spiritist Therapy. *Anthropologica* 35:23–38.

———. 1992. Spirits and Spiritist Therapy in Southern Brazil: A Case Study of an Innovative, Syncretic Healing Group. *Culture, Medicine and Psychiatry* 16:23–51.

———. 1991. Hypnosis and Trance Induction in the Surgeries of Brazilian Spirit Healer-mediums. *Anthropology of Consciousness* 2(3–4):20–25.

———. 1989. Pilgrimage, Therapy, and the Relationship between Healing and Imagination. Discussion Paper 82. Milwaukee: Center for Latin America, University of Wisconsin-Milwaukee.

———. 1987a. The Return of Dr. Fritz: Spiritist Healing and Patronage Networks in Urban, Industrial Brazil. *Social Science and Medicine* 24:1095–1108.

———. 1987b. "Romarias, Terapías, e a Ligação Entre as Curas e a Imagenação," In *Fé, Saúde, e Poder: Taumataurgos, Profetas, e Curandeiros.* Antonio Mourão Cavalcante, organizer, pp. 77–93. Fortaleza, Brazil: Centre de Cultura Popular de Canindé and Universidade Estadual do Ceará.

———. 1979a. Patron-Client Exchanges in Southeastern Minas Gerais. In *Brazil: Anthropological Perspectives. Essays in Honor of Charles Wagley.* M. Margolis and W. Carter, eds., pp. 362–78. New York: Columbia University Press.

——— 1979b. Plantations and Sugar Cane: An Historic and Developmental Overview. *Historical Reflections (Reflexions Historiques)* 6:85–119.

———. 1977a. Madeirà and the Beginnings of Sugar Cane Cultivation and Plantation Slavery: A Study in Institution Building. In *Comparative Perspectives in New World Plantation Societies.* Vera Rubin and Arthur Tuden, eds., pp. 536–52. Annals of the New York Academy of Sciences, no. 292. New York: New York Academy of Sciences.

———. 1977b. Patronage, Politics and the Articulation of Local Community and National Society in Pre-1968 Brazil. *Journal of Inter-American Studies and World Affairs* 19(2):139–72.

———. 1972. Charwomen, Cesspools and Road Building: An Examination of Patronage, Clientage and Political Power in Southeastern Minas Gerais. In *Structure and Process in Latin America: Patronage, Clientage and Power Systems.* A. Strickon and S. M. Greenfield, eds., pp. 71–199. Albuquerque: University of New Mexico Press.

Greenfield, Sidney M., and Antonio M. Cavalcante. 2006. Pilgrimage and Patronage in Brazil: A Paradigm for Social Relations and Religious Diversity. *Luso-Brazilian Review* 43(2):63–89.

Greenfield, Sidney M., and André Droogers. 2003. Syncretic Processes and the Definition of New Religions. *Journal of Contemporary Religion* 18(1):25–36.

References

Greenfield, Sidney M., and John Gray. 1989. *José Carlos and His Spirits: The Ritual Initiation of a Zelador dos Orixás.* Video documentary. Milwaukee: Educational Communications Department, University of Wisconsin-Milwaukee.

———. 1988. *The Return of Dr. Fritz: Healing by the Spirits in Brazil.* Video documentary. Milwaukee: Educational Communications Department, University of Wisconsin-Milwaukee.

———. 1985. *A Brazilian Pilgrimage: The "Festa de São Francisco" in Canindé.* Video documentary. Milwaukee: Educational Communications Department, University of Wisconsin-Milwaukee.

Greenfield, Sidney M., and Russel Prust. 1990. Popular Religion, Patronage, and Resource Distribution in Brazil: A Model of an Hypothesis for the Survival of the Economically Marginal. In *Perspectives on the Informal Economy.* M. E. Smith, ed., pp. 123–46. Lanham, MD: University Press of America.

Greenfield, Sidney M., and Arnold Strickon. 1981. A New Paradigm for the Study of Entrepreneurship and Social Change. *Economic Development and Cultural Change* 29(3):469–99.

Hall, Stephen S. 1999. All in the Timing: A Biologist Explores the Effect of Time on Humans and Science (review of *The Missing Moment: How the Unconscious Shapes Modern Science,* by Robert Pollack). *New York Times Book Review,* December 19, 28.

Harding, R. E. 2000. *A Refuge of Thunder: Candomblé and Alternative Spaces of Blackness.* Bloomington: Indiana University Press.

Harrington, Anne. 2008. *The Cure Within: A History of Mind-Body Medicine.* New York: W. W. Norton and Company.

Hervé, Ivan. 2006. *Reencarnação: A Única Explicação.* Porto Alegre, Brazil: Editora Age.

———. 2004. *Casa de João Pedro: Guia Para o Curso de Formação de Médiuns.* Porto Alegre, Brazil: Casa de João Pedro.

———. 1999. *Espiritualismo.* Porto Alegre, Brazil: Hércules.

———. 1996. *A Origem da Vida e Outras Origins.* Porto Alegre, Brazil: Editora Age.

Hervé, Ivan, Rogérion Sele da Silva, Volnei Borges, and Eva I. Tejada. 2003. *Apometria: A Conexão Entre a Ciência e o Espiritismo.* Porto Alegre, Brazil: Dacasa Editora/Livraria Palmerinca.

Hess, David J. 1993. *Science in the New Age: The Paranormal, Its Defenders and Debunkers, and American Culture.* Madison: University of Wisconsin Press.

——. n.d. Medical Pluralism in the Rhetoric of Encompassment: Four Religious Healing Systems in Brazil. Unpublished manuscript.

Hilgard, E. 1966. Posthypnotic Amnesia: Experiments and Theory. *International Journal of Clinical and Experimental Hypnosis* 14:104–11.

Holroyd, J. 1992. Hypnosis as a Methodology in Psychological Research. In *Contemporary Hypnosis Research*, E. Fromm and M. R. Nash, eds., pp. 210–26. New York: Guilford Press.

Hooneart, E. 1987. A Teologia das Romarias. *Diário do Nordeste*, October 11.

Hutchinson, B. 1966. The Patron-Dependent Relationship in Brazil: A Preliminary Examination. *Sociologia Ruralis* 6(1):3–30.

Inglis, Brian. 1989. *Trance: A Natural History of Altered States of Mind*. London: Grafton Books.

Isaacs, E. 1957. A History of American Spiritualism: The Beginnings, 1845–1855. Master's thesis, University of Wisconsin-Madison.

Kandel, Eric R. 1999. Biology and the Future of Psychoanalysis: A New Intellectual Framework for Psychiatry Revisited. *American Journal of Psychiatry* 156:505–24.

——. 1998. A New Intellectual Framework for Psychiatry. *American Journal of Psychiatry* 155:457–469.

Kardec, Allan. [1864] 1987. *The Gospel According to Spiritism*. J. Duncan, trans. English translation from the 3rd edition of the original French, published in 1866. London: Headquarters Publishing Co. Ltd.

——. [1861] 1975. *The Mediums' Book*. A. Blackwell, trans. São Paulo: Lake–Livraria Allan Kardec Editora Ltd.

——. [1857] n.d. *The Spirits' Book*. A. Blackwell, trans. São Paulo. Lake–Livraria Alan Kardec Editora Ltd.

Kendrick, Klaude. 1961. *The Promise Fulfilled: A History of the Modern Pentecostal Movement*. Springfield, MO: Gospel Publishing House.

Kent, Christopher. 2002. Placebo Surgery. *Chiropractic Journal*, September.

Kidder, Daniel P., and James C. Fletcher. 1857. *Brazil and the Brazilians, Portrayed in Historical and Descriptive Sketches*. Philadelphia: Childs and Peterson.

Klass, Morton. 1995. *Ordered Universes: Approaches to the Anthropology of Religion*. Boulder, CO: Westview Press.

Kleitman, Nathaniel. 1982. The Basic Rest-activity Cycle—22 Years Later. *Sleep* 5:311–15.

———. 1969. Basic Rest-Activity Cycle in Relation to Sleep and Wakefulness. In *Sleep, Physiology and Pathology*. Anthony Kales, ed., pp. 33–38. Philadelphia: Lippincott.

———. 1963. *Sleep and Wakefulness as Alternating Phases in the Cycle of Existence.* Chicago: University of Chicago Press.

Krippner, Stanley. 2008. *Learning from the Spirits: Candomble, Umbanda, and Kardecismo in Recife, Brazil.* Anthropology of Consciousness 19:1–32.

———. 2005. Trance and the Trickster: Hypnosis as a Liminal Phenomenon. *Journal of Clinical and Experimental Hypnosis* 523(2):97–118.

Kroeber, A. L. [1921] 1948. *Anthropology: Race, Language, Culture, Psychology, Prehistory.* New York: Harcourt, Brace and Co.

Kuhn, Thomas. 1970. *The Structure of Scientific Revolutions.* 2nd edition, enlarged. International Encyclopedia of Unified Science. Chicago: University of Chicago Press.

Lacerda de Azevedo, José. 1988. *Espirito/Matéria: Novos Horizontes para a Medecina.* Porto Alegre, Brazil: Pallotti.

Landes, Ruth. [1947] 1994. *City of Women.* Albuquerque: University of New Mexico Press.

Landim, Leilah. 1989. Quem São as "Seitas"? Sinais dos Tempos: Igrejas e Seitas no Brasil. *Cadernos do ISER* 21:11–21.

LeDoux, Joe. 2002. *Synaptic Self: How Our Brains Become Who We Are.* New York: Viking.

Lehmann, David.1996. *Struggle for the Spirit: Religious Transformation and Popular Culture in Brazil and Latin America.* Cambridge, MA: Blackwell Publishers.

LeShan, Lawrence. 1995. When Is Uvani? *Journal of the American Society for Psychical Research* 89:165–75.

Lévi-Strauss, Claude. 1966. *The Savage Mind.* Chicago: University of Chicago Press.

———. 1963. The Effectiveness of Symbols. In *Structural Anthropology*, vol. 1. Claire Jacobson and Brooke Grundfest Schoepf, trans., pp. 186–205. New York: Basic Books.

Lewontin, R. C., Steven Rose, and Leon K. Kamin. 1984. *Not in Our Genes: Biology, Ideology, and Human Nature.* New York: Pantheon Books.

Ley, R. G., and R. G. Freeman. 1984. Imagery, Cerebral Laterality, and the Healing Process. In *Imagination and Healing*. A. A. Sheikh, ed., pp. 51–68. Farmingdale, NY: Baywood.

Lloyd, David, and Ernest L. Rossi. 1992. *Ultradian Rhythms in Life Processes: A Fundamental Inquiry into Chronobiology and Psychobiology*. New York: Springer-Verlag.

Lohmann, Roger, ed. 2003. Perspectives on the Category "Supernatural." Special issue, *Anthropological Forum* 13.

Lowie, Robert. 1963. Religion in Human Life. *American Anthropologist* 65:532–42.

Lynch, D. W. 1996. Patient Satisfaction with Spiritist Healing in Brazil. Master's thesis, Department of Anthropology, University of Tennessee, Knoxville.

Machado, Maria das Dores C. 2003. Igreja Universal: Uma Organização Providência. In *Igreja Universal do Reino de Deus: Novos Conquistadors da Fé*. Ari Pedro Oro, André Corten, and Jean-Pierre Dozon, organizers, pp. 303–20. São Paulo: Editora Paulinas.

Maggie, Yvonnie. 1996. Aqueles a Quem foi Negado a Cor do Dia: As Categories Cor e Raça na Cultural Brasileira. In *Raça, Ciência e Sociedade*. Marcos C. Maio and Ricardo V. Santos, eds., pp. 225–34. Rio de Janeiro: Editora FIOCRUZ/CCBB.

Maio, Marcos C., and Ricardo V. Santos, organizers. 1996. *Raça, Ciência e Sociedade*. Rio de Janeiro: Editora FIOCRUZ/CCBB.

Mariano, Ricardo. 2003. O Reino da Propriedade da Igreja Universal. In *Igreja Universal do Reino de Deus: Novos Conquistadors da Fé*. Ari Pedro Oro, André Corten and Jean-Pierre Dozon, organizers, pp. 237–58. São Paulo: Editora Paulinas.

Mariz, Cecília Loreto. 1994. *Coping with Poverty: Pentecostals and Christian Base Communities in Brazil*. Philadelphia: Temple University Press.

Marmer, M. J. 1959. *Hypnosis in Anesthesiology*. Springfield, IL: Charles C. Thomas.

Mason, A., and A. Black. 1958. Allergic Skin Responses in Treatment of Asthma and Hay Fever by Hypnosis. *Lancet* 1:877–80.

Matthews, W. J., S. Lankton, and C. Lankton. 1993. An Eriksonian Model of Hypnosis. In *Handbook of Clinical Hypnosis*. J. W. Rhue, S. J. Lynn, and I. Kirsch, eds., pp. 187–214. Washington, DC: American Psychological Association.

References

McFague, Sallie. 1987. *Models of God: Theology for an Ecological, Nuclear Age.* Philadelphia: Fortress Press.

McGregor, Pedro. 1967. *Jesus of the Spirits.* New York: Stein and Day.

Mendonça, Antonio Gavea, and Procoro Velsques Filho. 1990. *Introdução ao Protestantismo no Brasil.* São Paulo: Loyola.

Merchant, K. 1996. *Pharmacological Regulation of Gene Expression in the CNS.* Boca Raton, FL: CRC Press.

Mesmer, Franz A. 1980. *Mesmerism: A Translation of the Original Scientific and Medical Writings of F. A. Mesmer.* George Bloch, translator and compiler. Los Altos, CA: William Kaufmann, Inc.

Milner, B., L. R. Squire, and E. R. Kandel. 1998. Cognitive Neuroscience and the Study of Memory. *Neuron* 20:445–68.

Moerman, D. E. 1979. Anthropology of Symbolic Healing. *Current Anthropology* 20:59–80.

Moore, Laurence E., and Jerold Z. Kaplan. 1983. Hypnotically Accelerated Burn Wound Healing. *American Journal of Clinical Hypnosis* 26:16–19.

Moore, Laurence R. 1977. *In Search of White Crows: Spiritualism, Parapsychology, American Culture.* New York: Oxford University Press.

Motta, Roberto. 2001. Ethnicity, Purity, the Market and Syncretism in Afro-Brazilian Cults. In *Reinventing Religions: Syncretism and Transformation in Africa and the Americas.* Sidney M. Greenfield and André Droogers, eds., pp. 71–85. Lanham, MD: Rowman and Littlefield.

———. 1998. Indian-Afro-European Syncretic Cults in Brazil: Their Economic and Social Roots. *Cahiers du Brésil Contemporain. Paris, Maison des sciences de L'Homme* 5:27–48.

———. 1982. Comida, Família, Dança e Transe: Sugessões Para o Estudo do Xangô. *Revista de Antropologia* (Universidade de São Paulo) 25:147–58.

Nagourney, E. 2001. A Study Links Prayer and Pregnancy. *New York Times,* October 2.

Nelson, Geoffrey K. 1969. *Spiritualism and Society.* London: Routlege and K. Paul.

Nørretranders, T. 1998. *The User Illusion: Cutting Consciousness Down to Size,* Jonathan Sydenham, trans. New York: Viking.

Orne, M. 1959. The Nature of Hypnosis: Artifact and Essence. *Journal of Abnormal and Social Psychology* 58:277–99.

Oro, Ari Pedro. 1999. *Axê Mercosur: As Religiões Afro-Brasileiros nos Países do Prata*. Petrópolis, Brazil: Editora Vozes.

———. 1988. Negros e Brancos nas Religiões AfroBrasileiros no Rio Grande do Sul. *Communicações do ISER* 7:33–54.

Osherson S., and L. AmaraSingham. 1981. The Machine Metaphor in Medicine. In *Social Contexts of Health, Illness and Patient Care*. E. Mishler, L. AmaraSingham, S. Hauser, R. Liem, S. Osherson, and N. Waxler, eds., pp. 218–49. Cambridge, England: Cambridge University Press.

Peacocke, A. R. 1979. *Creation and the World of Science*. Oxford: Clarendon Press.

Pert, Candace. 1997. *Molecules of Emotion: Why You Feel the Way You Feel*. New York: Scribner.

Pert, C., M. Ruff, R. Weber, and M. Herkenham. 1985. Neuropeptides and Their Receptors: A Psychosomatic Network. *Journal of Immunology* 135(2):820s–826s.

Pessar, Patricia R. 2004. *From Fanatics to Folk: Brazilian Millenarianism and Popular Culture*. Durham, NC: Duke University Press.

Pierucci, A. F., and R. Prandi. 1996. *A Realidade Social das Religiões no Brasil*. São Paulo: HUCITEC.

Pike, Kenneth L. 1967. *Language in Relation to a Unified Theory of the Structure of Human Behavior*. 2nd edition. The Hague: Mouton.

Polanyi, Karl, Conrad M. Arensberg, and Harry Pearson. 1957. *Trade and Market in the Early Empires: Economies in History and Anthropology*. Glencoe, IL: Free Press.

Prandi, Reginaldo. 1996. Religião Paga, Conversão e Serviço. *Novos Estudos* 45:65–77.

———. 1991. *Os Candomblés de São Paulo—A Velha Magia na Metrópole Nova*. São Paulo: HUCITEC-EDUSP.

Pressel, Esther. 1974. Umbanda, Trance and Possession in São Paulo, Brazil. In *Trance, Healing and Hallucination: Three Field Studies in Religious Experience*. F. D. Goodman, J. H. Henny, and E. Pressel, eds., pp. 113–26. New York: John Wiley and Sons.

Queiroz, Maria Isaoura Perreira de. 1973. *O Campesinato Brasileiro*. Petróplis, Brazil: Editora Vozes.

Quinn, Naomi. 1991. The Cultural Basis of Metaphor. In *Beyond Metaphor: The Theory of Tropes in Anthropology*. James Fernandez, ed., pp. 56–93. Stanford, CA: Stanford University Press.

References

Quinn, Naomi, and Dorothy Holland, eds. 1987. *Cultural Models in Language and Thought.* Cambridge: Cambridge University Press.

Randi, James A. 2005. *The ABC-TV Infomercial for John of God,* James Randi Educational Foundation, February 18, http://randi.org/jr/021805a.html#1

Flim-flam: Psychics, ESP, Unicorns and Other Delusions. Buffalo, NY: Prometheus Books.

Read, William. 1965. *New Patterns of Church Growth in Brazil.* Grand Rapids, MI: William B. Eerdmans.

Renshaw, Park. 1969. A Sociological Analysis of Spiritism in Brazil. PhD dissertation, University of Florida, Gainesville.

Rodgers, Denise. 2006. Mind-Body Modalities. In *Complementary and Integrative Medicine.* 3rd edition. Marc S. Micozzi, eds., pp. 280–312. St. Louis, MO: Saunders Elsiver.

Roniger, L. 1990. *Hierarchy and Trust in Modern Mexico and Brazil.* New York: Praeger.

———. 1987. Caciquismo and Coronelismo: Contextual Dimensions of Patron Brokerage in Mexico and Brazil. *Latin American Research Review 22*:71–99.

Rossi, Ernest L. 2002. *The Psychobiology of Gene Expression: Neuroscience and Neurogenesis in Hypnosis and the Healing Arts.* New York: W. W. Norton.

———. 2001. The Deep Psychobiology of Psychotherapy. In *Handbook of Innovative Therapy.* 2nd edition. R. Corsini, ed., pp. 155–65. New York: Wiley.

———. 1998. Mindbody Healing In Hypnosis: Immediate-early Genes and the Deep Psychobiology of Psychotherapy. *Japanese Journal of Hypnosis* 43:1–10.

———. [1986] 1993. *The Psychobiology of Mind-Body Healing: New Concepts of Therapeutic Hypnosis.* Revised edition. New York: W. W. Norton.

Rossi, Ernest L., and Kathryn L. Rossi. 1996. *The Symptom Path to Enlightenment: The New Dynamics of Self-organization in Hypnotherapy: An Advanced Manual for Beginners.* Pacific Palisades, CA: Palisades Gateway Publishing.

Ruzyla-Smith, P., A. Barabaz, M. Barabaza, and D. Warner. 1995. Effects of Hypnosis on the Immune Response: B-cells, T-cells, Helper and Supressor Cells. *American Journal of Clinical Hypnosis* 38:71–79.

Santos, Milton. 1993. *A Urbanizção Brasileira.* São Paulo: Editora HUCITEC.

Soares, Silvio Brito. 1962. *Vida e Obra de Bezerra de Menezes.* 7th edition. Rio de Janeiro: Federação Espírita Brasileira.

Star Online. 2008. "Brazil Raises Minimum Wage by 9 Per Cent." http://biz.thestar.com.my/news/story.asp?sec=business&file=/2008/3/2/business/20080302075622.

St. Clair, David. 1971. *Drum and Candle*. Garden City, NY: Doubleday and Company.

Steele, E. J., R. A. Lindley, and R.V. Blanden. 1998. *Lamarck's Signature: How Retrogenes Are Changing Darwin's Natural Selection Paradigm*. Reading, MA: Perseus Books.

Stoller, Paul. 1996. Sounds and Things: Pulsations of Power in Songhay. In *The Performance of Healing*, C. Laderman and M. Roseman, eds., pp. 165–84. New York: Routledge.

Strauss, C., and N. Quinn. 1994. A Cognitive/cultural Anthropology. In *Assessing Cultural Anthropology*, R. Borofsky, ed., pp. 284–300. New York: McGraw-Hill.

Tarnas, Richard. 1991. *The Passion of the Western Mind: Understanding the Ideas That Have Shaped Our World View*. New York: Ballantine.

Trindade, D. F. 1989. *Iniciação à Umbanda*. 2nd edition. São Paulo: Tríade Editora, Ltda.

Trölle, T. R., J. Schadrack, and W. Zieglgänsberger. 1995. Preface. In *Immediate-early Genes in the Central Nervous System*, by J. Schadrack and W. Zieglgänsberger. Berlin: Springer.

Tully, T. 1996. Discovery of Genes Involved with Learning and Memory: An Experimental Synthesis of Hirschian and Benzerian Perspectives. *Proceedings of the National Academy of Sciences of the United States of America* 93:13460–67.

Turner, Victor. 1987, 1988. *The Anthropology of Performance*. 1st edition. NY: PAJ Publications.

———. [1964] 1979. Betwixt and Between: The Liminal Period in *Rites de Passage*. In *Reader in Comparative Religion: An Anthropological Approach*. 4th edition. W. Lessa and E. Vogt, eds., pp. 234–43. New York: Harper and Row.

———. 1969. *The Ritual Process: Structure and Anti-structure*. Chicago: Aldine.

———. 1968. Myth and Symbol. In *International Encyclopedia of the Social Sciences*, D. L. Sills, ed., vol. 10, pp. 576–82. New York: Macmillan/Free Press.

———. 1967. *The Forest of Symbol: Aspects of Ndembu Ritual*. Ithaca, New York: Cornell University Press.

Tylor, Edward B. [1871] 1958. *Primitive Culture, vol. 1: The Origins of Culture*. New York: Harper and Brothers.

References

Verger, Pierre. 1976. *Trade Relations between the Bight of Benin and Bahia from the 17th to the 19th Centuries.* Ibadan: Ibadan University Press.

————. 1964. *Bahia and the West Coast Trade.* Ibadan: University of Ibadan Press.

Wafer, Jim. 1991. *The Taste of Blood: Spirit Possession in Brazilian Candomblé.* Philadelphia: University of Pennsylvania Press.

Weisberg, Barbara. 2004. *Talking to the Dead: Kate and Maggie Fox and the Rise of Spiritualism.* San Francisco: Harper San Francisco.

Wells, H. G. [1899] 2000. *When the Sleeper Wakes.* L. Stover, ed. Jefferson, NC: McFarland.

Westmeier, Karl-Wilhelm. 1999. *Protestant Pentecostalism in Latin America: A Study in the Dynamics of Missions.* Cranbury, NJ: Associated University Presses.

Williams, Mary W., Ruhl J. Bartless, and Russell E. Miller. 1955. *The People and Politics of South America.* Boston: Ginn and Company.

Wilson, Stephen, ed. 1983. *Saints and Their Cults: Studies in Religious Sociology, Folklore and History.* Cambridge, England: Cambridge University Press.

Winkelman, Michael. 2000. *Shamanism: The Neural Ecology of Consciousness and Healing.* Westport, CT: Bergin and Garvey.

————. 1997. Altered States of Consciousness and Religious Behavior. In *Anthropology of Religion: A Handbook.* S. D. Glazier, ed., pp. 393–428. Westport, CT: Greenwood Press.

Wolf, Eric. 1974. *Anthropology.* New York: Norton.

Woodward, Kenneth L. 1990. *Making Saints: How the Catholic Church Determines Who Becomes a Saint, Who Doesn't, and Why.* New York: Touchstone.

Xavier, Francisco Candido. 1944. Nosso Lar. Dictated by the spirit André Luiz. Rio de Janeiro: Federação Espírita Brasileira.

Zimmermann, Manfred. 1989. The Nervous System in the Context of Information Theory. In *Human Physiology.* 2nd edition. R. F. Schmidt and G. Thews, eds., pp. 166–73. Berlin: Springer.

————. 1986. Neurophysiology of Sensory Systems. In *Fundamentals of Sensory Physiology.* R. F. Schmidt, ed., pp. 68–116. Berlin: Springer.

INDEX

Note: Italicized page numbers indicate illustrations.

Index

Index

magnetic healing, 181
Malù (Maria de Lourdes Nardi), 59–60
Marco Antônio. *See* Santos, Marco Antônio dos
Maria Laura (cousin of Maria da Fatima Batista), 105
Maria Laura (radio show hostess), 33, 36
Maria Padilha *(exu)*, 131–33
Maria (Italian immigrant convert to Afro-Brazilian religion), 122–23
Mariz, Cecília, 146
Marta (sister-in-law of Anna), 83, 84
Mason, Arthur, 182
material body, relationship of spirit with, 82
material plane, 69, 71
Mauricio. *See* Magalhães, Mauricio
McPherson, Aimee Semple, 139
Mead, Margaret, 11
meaning systems, symbolic, 13–14
mechanistic vs. organic model of the world, 166
medical anthropology, 47, 167, 171, 180, 212 n52
medical sciences, 68, 159–60, 165, 167, 171
medications prescribed by Spiritist healer-mediums, 27–30
Mediterranean rules of city-founding, 138–39
mediums, 24, 28, 74, 88, *124*. *See also* Spiritist healer-mediums
Medium's Book, The (Kardec), 38
Mello, Manoel de, 139–40
memory and learning, 169, 175–77, 180, 191
mental illness, 73–74
mesa branca (white table), 84
Mesmer, Franz Anton, 55, 181
Mesmer Society of Paris, 55–56
metaphor, in representations of world view, 164
migrants, rural, 150
mindbody communication, psychobiological arousal and, 191–92
mind/body dualism, 160, 161, 171
minimum wage (in Brazil), 148–49
Miranda, David, 140
missionaries, 96, 136, 138–40
models, as basis for understanding, 163–64
Morais, Zélio de, 125–27
morality, as defined by Spiritists, 38
multinational corporations in Brazil, 148
music, in rituals, 128–30, 179–80, 196, 198
mythological themes, in rituals, 178

Nagô language, 120
Nardi, Maria de Lourdes (Malù), 59
National Evangelization Crusade, 139
National Health Services offices, 33
natural/supernatural dichotomy, 156, 158–60
nature and nurture interaction, 170, 172–73
needles, in healing, 61–63
Neo-Europe concept, 101
neo-Pentecostal churches, 141–43
neuropeptides and neuropeptide receptors, 210–11 n40
neuroscience, and culturalbiological imagery, 172–73
Niteroi, Brazil, 125
nondeclarative memory and learning, 175
nonwhites, in Brazil, 126
normal waking state vs. altered states of consciousness, 185
Nosso Lar (publication), 70–71

Obaluaé/St. Lazarus, 130
obsession, Kardec's use of term, 73–74
Ogun/St. George, 76, 130
organic model of the world, 166
organic vs. mechanistic model of the world, 166
orientation sessions, 90
orixás/saints, as protectors, 130
Ouija boards, 48

Pai Joaquim *(preto velho)*, 131, 134
pais-de-santo (fathers in sainthood), 121
Palmelo, Brazil, *8* (map), 50, *56*
pantomimed surgeries, 77
paradigms, 165–66
paranormal, meaning of, 155–56
parapsychology, 155
parasympathetic dominant state and relaxation response, 189–90
Parham, Charles P., 208 n27
passes, in Spiritist healings, 28, 68, 77, 86
pastors, in Brazil, 138–39
patients: ailments of, treated by Mauricio Magalhães/Dr. Fritz, 60–61; altered states of consciousness of, 88; benefits of Spiritist healings to, 57; demographics of, 80, 206 n13; experience following disobsession, 88; experiences during disobsession ritual, 79, 82; experiences during surgery, 46, 52, 54, 62–63; listening to testimonials, *192*; previous lives of, in diagnosis and treatment, 74–75; recovery of, 55; response to surgeries, 43; survey of, 58–63; in trancelike state, 53, 89, *192*

Index

Roman Catholic Church, 96. *See also* Catholicism

romeiros (pilgrims), 104, 199

Rossi, Ernest L., 18, 168–70, 187–89, 191–92

sacrifices, of animals, 132–33

saints: reciprocity in relationships between petitioners and, 107

saints, in Brazil, 106, 108, 130, 207 n20

Santos, Celestina de Araujo, 127–29, 133–34, 145–47, 198

Santos, Marco Antônio dos, 129, 131–34

São Francisco das Chagas (St. Francis of the Wounds), 104

São Francisco de Chagas in Candindé, *114–15*

saw, electric, as surgical tool, 51

Schadrack, J., 166

Schutz, Paulo, 15, 65–72

Schutz, Sueli, 68, 71, 72

science and sciences: Cartesian, 158–59; as cultural process, 17–18, 163; improbability in, 157; medical, 68, 165, 167; modern, 157–59; neuroscience, 172–73; proof of value in, 87; reformulation of, in healing process, 162

scientific communities, 164, 165

séances, 48

Sergio (pilgrim), 112–13

serial logic, 175–76

Seymour, William Joseph, 136–37

shrines to saints, 105, 107, 114

sinus problems, treatment for, 45

slaves and slavery, in Brazil, 11, 96–97, 99, 117–19

social anthropology, cardinal sin of, 156

social categories in Brazilian history, 130–31

social groups, and symbolic categories, 173

sociobiology, 172

Southern Baptist Convention, 136

Spain, and Treaty of Tordesilhas, 95

spinal surgery, 12

spirit beings, as functional concepts, 160

spirit doctors, 51, *56*, 74–75. *See also* Fritz, Dr. Adolph; St. Ignatius of Loyola; Stams, Dr. Ricardo

Spiritism: in continuum of Brazilian religions, 84; and coping with death and dying, 30, 72; as ethic of practical charity, 38; growth of, 141; lectures on, in testimonials, 194–96; as morally driven system of beliefs, 70; origins of, 37–38, 99

Spiritist centers: at Niteroi, 125; at Recife,

35–48, 89, 193–96; at Rio de Janeiro, 75–79

Spiritist Federation, 30, 39, 48

Spiritist healer-mediums: diagnosis by, 74; hypnosis denial by, 197; and illness, 69; in Kardecism, 28; licensed physicians and, 30–31, 36–37, 40; medications prescribed by, 27–30; prescription writing by, 43; success of treatments by, 87; and theater metaphor, 197. *See also* Spiritist healings; Spiritist surgeries

Spiritist healings: benefits to patients, 57; as charity, 80; enlightened spirits and, 74; and getting at the source, 46–47; passes in, 28, 68, 77, 86; scientific proof of value, 87; testimonials and, 75–76

Spiritist movement, 61

Spiritist publications, 70–71

Spiritists. *See* Kardecist-Spiritists

Spiritist surgeries: breast, 12, 35–36; at a distance, 194; eye, 12, 23–26; growth removal, 43; for impacted arteries, 53–55; lectures and testimonials as prelude to, 194–96; to let spirits do their work, 49, 57, 62; for old bullet wound, 50–51; performed by Edson Querioz/Dr. Fritz, *40–41, 40*–43; purpose of, 91–92; spinal, 12; success of, in survey findings, 61; and theater metaphor, 196; witnessed by author, 47. *See also* patients

Spirit of the Seven Crossroads *(Caboclo das Sete Encruzilhadas),* 125

spirit plane, 70–71

spirit possessions: compared to hypnotically facilitated trance, 199; continuation of African practice of, 118; by deceased doctors and healers, 75; of Edson Queiroz, 40; of José Carlos Ribeiro, 23–24, 30; of Mãe Edna, 132; of Marc Antônio, 134

spirits: African-derived, 84; communication with, 37–38; developmental path of, 69–70; free will of, 38; interventions with, 87; malevolent, 85; and mediums, 24; and mental illness, 73–74; non-European, 125; Pentecostals and, 141–42; rehabilitation for, 74; relationship of material body with, 82; relationships and groups of, 71; of Umbanda, 83, 125, 131

Spirits' Book, The (Kardec), 38

spirit stories of Brazilians, 145–46

St. Francis, pilgrims' vows to, 104, 111–13, *114–15*

St. Francis of Assisi Festival *(Festa de São Francisco),* Candindé, 103–4, 109–14

237

Index

St. Francis of the Wounds *(São Francisco das Chagas)*, 104
St. Ignatius of Loyola, 25, 205 n4
Stams, Dr. Ricardo, 51, *56*. *See also* Rios, Antonio de Oliveira/Dr. Stams
state-dependent memory, learning, behavior (SDMLB), 169, 176–77, 191
stress, and depressed immune function, 169–70
structural concepts, 160
Structure of Scientific Revolutions, The (Kuhn), 163–66
sugar, and slavery in Brazil, 96–97
supernatural beings: African deities, 76, 83, 97–98, 206–7 n15; and assistance for injuries and illnesses, 111; Catholicism and, 158; connection to, in West Africa, 118; deities of Umbanda, 130–31; range of, available to Brazilians, 147. *See also* spirits
surgeries, 49, 77, 205 n3. *See also* Spiritist surgeries
surgical instruments, 27, 51, *56*
survey of patients treated by Mauricio Magalhães/Dr. Fritz, 58–63
surveys in U.S., 60
symbolic information, transmission of, 173–74
symbolic meaning systems, 13–14
symbolism, in representations of world view, 163
symbols, 173, 177–78
syringe needles, use by Mauricio Magalhães/Dr. Fritz, 61–63

table turning, 48
Tavares, Levy, 140
tax burden in Brazil, 149–50
Teixeira, Cícero Marcos, 65–66, 68
Teixeira de Farias, João (John of God), 44, 205 n4
television, use by evangelists, 143
terpsichoretrance, 184
terreiros, 120–22
testimonials, 75–76, 90, 190–91, *192*, 194–96
theater metaphor, and surgery, 197
tithing, 142–43
tongues, talking in, 136–37
trances: in Brazilian healing practices, 184–85; common everyday, 187; defined, 183; hypnotically facilitated, 18, 195, 199; patients in, 53, 89, *192*; religious, 186
transduction, 211 n41
treatment at a distance, 67
Treaty of Tordesilhas, 95

triage, 194
Trölle, T. R., 174
Turner, Victor, 178, 198
Tylor, Sir Edward B., 13, 157, 172

ultradian rhythms of waking and sleeping, *188*
Umbanda: and 1960s counterculture movement, 121; *Casa de Vovô Maria*, 127–28; case descriptions, 127–34; in continuum of Brazilian religions, 84; deities of, 130–31; growth of, 141; Zélio de Morais and, 126–27; origins of, 99; race of followers, 208 n24; rituals of, 129; spirits of, 83, 125; syncretism of, 206–7 n15; theology of, 130
Umbral, 85
unemployment rate in Brazil, 149
Universal Church of the Kingdom of God *(Igreja Universal do Reino de Deus)* (IURD), 141–43, 199
UN Millenium Project, 150
Uvani, 160

Vingren, Gunnar, 137
votive offerings, *114–15*

Wagley, Charles, 11
wave nature of consciousness and being, 186–89
wealth and poverty in Brazil, 148–50
wealth in Brazil, 210 n34
Weber, Max, 13
Wells, H. G., 203
Wesley, John, 208 n26
West Africa, 118, 119, 198–99
When the Sleeper Awakes (Wells), 203
whitening of Brazil's population, 126
white table *(mesa branca)*, 84
Williams, Harold, 139
Winkelman, Michael, 189–90
woman offering her hair as a votive offering, *114–15*
World Bank, and economy of Brazil, 148
world views, 163–64, 166, 177–78

Xangô religion, 83, 84
Xangô/St. Jerome, 129

yoga, 52

Zé Arigó, 26, 32
Zieglgänsberger, W., 166
Zimmerman, Manfred, 174

ABOUT THE AUTHOR

Sidney M. Greenfield, Professor of Anthropology Emeritus at the University of Wisconsin-Milwaukee, has conducted ethnographic research in the West Indies and New Bedford, Massachusetts and, since 1959, anthropologically oriented research in Brazil. He also has done ethnohistory and historical research in Portugal and the Atlantic Islands, studying problems ranging from family and kinship, patronage and politics, the history of plantations and plantation slavery and entrepreneurship to Spiritist surgery and healing and syncretized Brazilian religions. Greenfield has received numerous research grants and four Fulbright awards that have enabled him to serve as a Visiting Professor at three Brazilian Universities. His latest projects include a study of the participation of Evangelical Protestants in politics in Brazil, the distribution of income and wealth and ways to reduce inequality and poverty. Author and/or editor of seven books, producer, director and author of five video documentaries, he has published some 130 chapters in books, articles and reviews in professional journals. He lives in New York City where he is co-chair of the Columbia University Seminar on Brazil. His e-mail address is: sgreenfield222@aol.com